Christian
Caregiving

DR. WILLIAM E. HULME

Christian Caregiving

*Insights from the
Book of Job*

▼

Publishing House
St. Louis

Copyright © 1992 Concordia Publishing House
3558 S. Jefferson Avenue, St. Louis, MO 63118-3968
Manufactured in the United States of America

Library of Congress Cataloging-in-Publication Data

Hulme, William Edward, 1920–
    Christian caregiving: insights from the Book of Job/William E. Hulme.
      p.   cm.
    ISBN 0-570-04564-9
    1. Pastoral counseling. 2. Bible. O.T. Job—Criticism, interpretation, etc. I. Title.
  BV4012. 2. H799 1992
  253.5—dc20
                                   91-33156

1 2 3 4 5 6 7 8 9 10   01 00 99 98 97 96 95 94 93 92

CONTENTS

745

119650

INTRODUCTION

The multidimensional nature of the content and style of Job has fascinated theologians, literary scholars, and lay Bible readers during the millennia since it was composed. As a pastoral theologian, the book's profundity in divine wisdom and insight into the human spirit has long amazed me and ministered to me. I have chosen to focus primarily on two of aspects of its diverse nature which contain this divine wisdom and insight into the human condition.

The first dimension is the threat that suffering presents to our sense of meaning and justice and to any joy in living. This threat is depicted within the setting of counseling relationships between Job, his friends, and God. This setting is the basis for the second dimension, namely, the wisdom and insight into the ministry of spiritual counseling that is revealed in the dynamics of these relationships. These dimensions are intrinsically related and provide us with the church's own indigenous resource for its counseling and caring ministry.

1. A Root of Contemporary Pastoral Counseling

In his book *Roots and Shoots* (London: Hodder and Stoughton, 1985), Roger F. Hurding traces the roots and shoots of the contemporary pastoral counseling ministry. The roots are the various schools of psychotherapy that have been evolving since Freudian psychoanalysis. What is missing in Hurding's "tree of healing" is any root in the Bible itself. He refers to using the Bible in pastoral counseling, but not to any source or root in the Bible for pastoral counseling. The Book of Job is precisely such a root.

Many schools of psychotherapy have contributed to what

is now known as the ministry of pastoral counseling. They focus on their own specific understanding of the human psyche and the ways to meet its needs. But contrary to what most of these schools assert, they have not discovered anything really new. What each has done is to *re*discover in a contemporary culture some specific foci of intuitive wisdom that have been known previously by ancient healers. In our contemporary society, the innovative psychotherapist has utilized the Western scientific method and the relatively new human science of psychology to research, clarify, and systematize a portion of ancient wisdom.

The counseling process in the Book of Job is perceived largely by induction. The communications are presented as poetic speeches in which each participant takes his turn in poetic symmetry. In spite of this literary format—or perhaps *through* this literary format—the dynamics of the counseling encounter are remarkably presented.

Most studies of the Book of Job are conducted by Old Testament scholars, exegetes, and literary scholars. I am not in any of these categories. What my eyes have been trained to see and my ears to hear as a pastoral theologian and counselor may be different from that perceived by scholars in these other branches of theological study. We need all branches together for a balanced perspective of the biblical texts. I have read the Old Testament commentaries and treatises on the Book of Job and profited much from them. While I am not proficient in the Hebrew language of the Old Testament, I have studied Hebrew and can follow the writings of those who have this expertise. I will utilize the knowledge of these scholars in this book. I particularly appreciate the work of Samuel Terrien of Yale University whose knowledge of language and literary research is combined with a keen pastoral perspective. In contrast to many scholars Terrien sees the value of the Elihu portion of the book, whose contribution is almost exclusively pastoral (*Job, Poet of Existence*, New York: Bobbs-Merrill, 1957; also The Interpreters Bible, Vol. 3 [Job]).

It may seem presumptuous or even naive to perceive a modern understanding of Christian counseling in this ancient document. But this assumption of presumption or naivete would be based on the illusion (which, as I have noted, is widely held) that pastoral and counseling wisdom is a Western—perhaps even American—and a modern-day discovery. The reality is that what we now perceive as pastoral wisdom is actually the God-given wisdom of the ages. My task in this book is simply to elucidate the spiritual counseling significance of these poetic speeches as they relate to each other in terms of our contemporary awareness. In so doing I will be highlighting a biblical base—a root—for Christian care and counseling that is prior to any indebtedness of Christian counseling to the insights of modern (and western) psychotherapy.

I will focus on the dynamics that are implicit—and often explicit—in these speeches in Job. What is going on emotionally between the counselors and the counselee? What are the relational dynamics that are perceptible to a counseling-trained reader? The book of Job is structured around these dynamics. Our own experiences, particularly with pain, help us perceive these dynamics. The relationships between Job and his counselors as well as between Job and God are emotionally charged. Consequently, an emotional perception is needed along with an intellectual perception to perceive what is transpiring in these supposedly therapeutic encounters.

The theories of the authorship of Job run the gamut from the prior existence of the prologue and epilogue and subsequent addition of the poetic section, to the prior existence of the poetic section and the subsequent addition of the prologue and epilogue, to the view that the poetic author was the one who later wrote the prologue and epilogue.

Since these are all theories lacking firsthand knowledge, we obviously cannot be dogmatic about the origins of the book. What we can say with assurance is that all of the parts of the book hold together remarkably well. Even the Elihu portion, which some scholars believe to be a later addition to the poetic section, is precisely where it belongs from a counselor perspective. Though Elihu is not mentioned in either the poetic section with the three friends or in the prologue or epilogue, his contribution is the needed psychological and spiritual bridge from the defiant Job, at the conclusion of his counseling by the three friends, to the theophany and the subsequently receptive Job, who is changed from within. Also, the content of the prologue enters repeatedly into the poetic section. In fact, the prologue is the implicit backdrop in the poetic section's search for a livable theodicy—a way to live harmoniously with the love and justice of God, and with the tragedies, sufferings, and evils of this world. Some believe that the integration of all of these parts is due to an editor rather than the original writer or writers.

The theodicy of the prologue may seem strange to us modern Westerners who have difficulty grasping the significance of Eastern stories. Yet what theodicy is not strange when viewed from a different perspective? The fact is that the search for a theodicy is doomed by the very nature of its quest not to find any universal acceptance. In any theodicy, the information or picture that is presented pertains to a mystery. Yet the human mind needs a framework, upon which to contemplate the mystery. But the theodicy, whether Eastern or Western, ancient or modern, does not fully resolve the mystery; it only helps us to live with it.

2. Empathy with or Resistance to Pain

Because it is centered in interpersonal dynamics, spiritual counseling may be threatening to both the counselor and the counselee. This is clearly revealed in the Book of Job. The three comforter-counselors were offended by Job's expression of despair and were unwilling or unable to enter into the depths of his feelings. But when one has the compassion to go with another into the depths of emotional sharing, the involvement affects both spiritual counselor and counselee. As sufferers reveal their souls to one who is open to receive, they clarify for themselves what is going on within them.

Spiritual counselors who allow themselves to enter into the emotional pain of their counselees will grow in their own self-knowledge as well. Obviously, it takes more than knowledge to become effective as a spiritual counselor; it also takes self-knowledge and courage.

As the suffering Job bares his soul for all to see in the poetic section, the reader can empathize with the frustration and despair that suffering engenders. This identification is the initial spiritual counselor response to the counselee, which in turn influences what the counselor *says* to the sufferer—or does *not* say. It is my intention to elucidate these two counseling-oriented dimensions contained in the Book of Job—the affective description of the sufferer in the throes of pain and the response of the counselor to this expression of pain—as each relates to the other.

The picture of the one in pain described in the book may seem most extreme. The difference between Job's experience of pain and loss and that of others, however, is only one of degree and not of kind. In fact, some sufferers may identify with Job precisely because they too have been hit with one loss after another. Even when this is not the case, one's own pain may *seem* like Job's in terms of its effect on oneself.

For this reason it is unwise for a counselor to minimize the counselee's troubles. While they may appear to be relatively minimal to the observer, they are enormous to the sufferer. Why should this be? Again, it is the effect of the trauma on the sufferer that helps determine the pain. Its effect is horrendous to the degree that it threatens the person's perspective of living. How important for one's sense of worth and hence, one's reason for living, is that which has been lost—or threatened with loss? Because of this relativity of the *effect,* it is really not strange when the counselor's attempt to reassure a person that his/her problem is really not that big—does not reassure. In fact, it may convince the counselee of the counselor's inability to understand.

On the other hand, when one can allow oneself to feel the pain of the other—even though one may not understand

11

why it should be so severe—one is in position to tap one's intuitive wisdom in responding. It is the picture of suffering which the Book of Job so powerfully portrays that stimulates the compassion that assists one to counsel. As Henri Nouwen puts it, "The beginning of healing is in the solidarity with the pain" (*Reaching Out*, New York: Doubleday, 1975, p. 43).

Concurrent with this picture of the sufferer are the responses to it—from the three friends and from Elihu. In addition, there is Job's own counsel to his friends concerning how to respond to his pain. Unfortunately, they did not or could not receive his counsel. Their own resistance to the threat of Job's expression set them in a defensive position in which they could no longer receive.

When we are threatened, we are frightened. Only courage can move us to receive when we are frightened. It is also courage that is needed to utilize our own intuitive wisdom. How does one acquire this courage? The very nature of Christian counseling implies the presence of the divine Counselor—the awareness of whose presence gives the Christian counselor the perspective and the courage to do what self-awareness alone may not.

But the route to our capacity for compassion and wisdom is blocked by more than our fear. We are products of a culture which pressures us to compete and achieve in order to establish and affirm our worth. The loneliness of the competer can overtake even the counselor. When this is the case, one's stance is largely defensive, and protecting oneself overrides the desire to risk oneself. Allowing oneself to feel the pain of the other is a risk. Can we handle it? Better not to expose ourselves to that question! How then does one decondition oneself from cultural conditioning?

The methodology of counseling, based on the wisdom of the ages as revealed in the Book of Job, can, when practiced, be a step in the direction of cultural deconditioning. Who we are (our being) affects our behavior (our doing), and our doing also contributes in turn to our being. So there can be a continuously mutual interaction between our being and our doing. Just learning to say the right words in our response can lead us into the emotional atmosphere that will take us past our protective roadblocks.

Yet even methodology can be distorted for our own protection. In *The Wounded Healer* Henri Nouwen presents the verbatim of a student chaplain (John) with a hospital patient (Mr. Harrison) facing surgery, in which the patient gives all kinds of clues to his inner crisis. Because the student had been taught the right way to respond, he was not oblivious to what he should do when he heard the clues. But to do so would have evidently created his own inner crisis. So he worded his restatement of the patient's clues in such a generalized way that he could avoid dealing with the pain. He used his knowledge of method to protect himself by a careful use of words that neutralized the threat. The following excerpt illustrates his deftness in blunting his responses.

Referring to the patient's approaching operation, the chaplain asked, "You feel ready for it?"

Mr. Harrison: "Well, I'm not ready to die. But I think the operation is necessary, or I'll lose my legs."

John: "You're not ready for the end, but you want something to be done if possible so you won't lose your legs."

Mr. Harrison: "Yeah (nodding). If this is the end, this is one who's gonna be lost."

John: "You feel the cause is lost if you don't make it through the operation" (Henri Nouwen, *The Wounded Healer,* New York: Image Books, 1979, p. 53).

In his first response, the chaplain substituted the word "end" for "die," and in the second, he substituted the word "cause" for the patient himself. In each instance, he avoided dealing not only with the patient's obvious fear of dying but also with the patient's fear of eternal judgment.

Responses such as this student chaplain's, by a careful selection of words, seem to fulfill the letter of the methodology but certainly violate the spirit because they bypass the emotional pain in the counselee's communication. In their generalized formulation they lack specificity and precision and are intellectually rather than emotionally focused. Ironically, the intellectual focus is a defense against the counselor's own emotional (fear) reaction to the counselee's communication. Our intellect is often the unwitting defense system against our unfaced feelings.

3. A Difficult Text

In concentrating in the Book of Job on the experience of pain by the counselee and the responses of the counselors, we need to remind ourselves that we are dealing with a most difficult text. The poetry is of excellent literary quality, and it is not coincidental that one with such amazing sensitivity to the existential drama of intra- and interpersonal relationships is a poet. But this poet uses many words that are not found in other Hebrew writings of the day. The poet is an original thinker as well as a fine artist and perhaps deliberately chose words for their precision and beauty more than for their familiarity. But this provides a severe challenge for the translators. They are even more severely challenged since the text that has been handed down to us, through the continuous copying of the manuscript over many centuries, may not always have been well preserved. But it has been preserved, and for this we are grateful. It leaves, however, many instances where the translator must make an educated guess as to the meaning of a word or a grammatical structure.

Those places where the translators have made their educated guesses are carefully noted in the Revised Standard Version, which I will be using. I will attempt to avoid basing any insights into the counselee's inner dynamics or the counselor's responses on these obscure parts of the book. Fortunately, for most of the book, the translation is substantiated by the relatively clear Hebrew text. In those few instances where obscure texts are involved in my elucidation, I will attempt to defend my use of the translation.

In elucidating the wisdom for Christian counseling and caregiving that I perceive in the Book of Job, I shall follow the sequence of the book as we now have it, beginning with the prologue and concluding with the epilogue. The major focus, however, will be on the poetic sections: first, the speeches of Job and the three friends; second, the speeches of Elihu; and third, the encounter with God or the theophany.

Chapter One

When the Inner Becomes the Outer

In the prologue Job is presented as a very successful person. He was a man of the East, though the location of Uz is unknown. His success is his wealth: sheep, camels, oxen, she-asses, and the many servants to care for them. It is also his family: seven sons and three daughters. But it was primarily his character: "blameless and upright." "Blameless" (*tam*) means that one's conduct is free from objection—complete in the virtues extolled in biblical Wisdom literature. "Upright" refers to his social relationships: Job was honest, just, a person of great integrity. But the source for this successful life was his faith. Job "feared God, and turned away from evil" (1:1).

The only possible flaw in the picture is the description of Job's family. The children were very close in their relationships with each other. Though they evidently lived in their own dwellings in the regal manner fitting for adult children of a wealthy Eastern patriarch, they regularly gathered together for parties in each other's homes that lasted for days. But when these parties were over Job sacrificed burnt offerings on their behalf. "It may be that my sons have sinned, and cursed God in their hearts" (1:5). Here and throughout the poetic section Job understands religious devotion as not only focused in outward acts but also in inward attitudes. Evidently he was uneasy about what might have gone on in their "insides" during these festivities, and so he offererd sacrifice for their forgiveness. There is also a reference to Job's children in the poetic section that seems to substantiate Job's concern (8:4).

1. Theodicy—a Metaphysical Drama

This presentation of Job as the ultimate in human development through faith, however, was too much for Satan, the adversary. So he challenged God's affirmation of Job's character by asking, "Does Job fear God for nought?"(1:9). This question is an integrating theme for the poetic section as well. Elihu, for example, rewords it when he restates Job's question, "How am I better off than if I had sinned?" (35:3). The adversary charged that God had protected Job from the troubles of life—putting "a hedge about him and his house and all that he has, on every side" (1:10). Had this protection been the payoff for his faith in God—for his moral and spiritual uprightness? Find out! Take the blessings away—deprive him of his family and possessions and see what happens. Satan is quite sure of the outcome. Job "will curse thee to thy face" (1:11).

The idea of fearing God for nought contrasts with another line of thought in the Old Testament which emphasizes the rewards that come to those who fear God. If this seems to be a more primitive religious concept, it should be recalled that in the Old Testament, what happens after death is not as clearly defined as in the New Testament, with its focus on the Resurrection. In fact, Job grapples with this question in the poetic section more than once. If only a human death could be like that of a dead tree, he opined, then a new shoot could come from the stump and life could resume (14:7–10). He openly raises the question, "If a man die, shall he live again?" (14:14).

Job's three counselors applied the justice that goes with belief in God to life in this world. However, whether one looks to this life only, or also to a life beyond to vindicate God's justice in the universe, the nature of the reasoning is the same if faith expects a reward.

To fear God for nought is something other. It is to affirm with almost nonsensical loyalty that regardless of what God does, one will not only remain faithful but even bless God's name. St. Francis Xavier extended this idea even to eternity in his New Testament thinking:

Then why, O blessed Jesus Christ, Should I not love Thee well? Not for the sake of winning heaven, or of escaping hell; Not with the hope of gaining aught; Not seeking a reward; But as Thyself hast loved me, O ever-loving Lord. E'en so I love Thee, and will love, And in Thy praise will sing; Solely because Thou art my God, and my eternal King.[1]

St. Bernard of Clairvaux's four levels of love culminate also in a no-rewards motive: to love God solely for God's sake. This kind of love is a reflection of God's love, as expressed in Isaiah 43:25: "I am He who blots out your transgressions *for my own sake*, and I will not remember your sins" (italics added). There is also a similar Old Testament theme in terms of life in this world in the prophet Habbakuk:

Though the fig tree do not blossom, nor fruit be on the vines, the produce of the olive fail, and the fields yield no food, the flock be cut off from the fold, and there be no herd in the stalls, yet I will rejoice in the Lord, I will joy in the God of my salvation" (3:17–18).

In the metaphysical drama of the prologue, God accepts the adversary's challenge. Satan is given leave to test Job by afflicting him with all sorts of deprivations and losses. There is a symmetry to the description of the calamities. As each messenger of bad news told his story—the loss of the oxen and asses, then the sheep and the servants, followed by the camels and servants—the concluding words were, "and I alone have escaped to tell you" (1:19). But the biggest blow was yet to come—a great wind had struck the house where Job's children were partying and destroyed it, killing all ten of the children.

Quite a pileup! But this pileup does not necessarily separate Job from other sufferers. Their familiarity is shown in the aphorism, "It never rains but it pours."

---

[1] "My God, I Love Thee," transl. Edward Caswell, Hymn 80 in *The English Hymnal* (London: Oxford, 1933). Cf. "O God, I Love Thee," Hymn 491 in *Lutheran Book of Worship* (Minneapolis: Augsburg, 1978).

Overwhelmed by it all, Job rent his robe and shaved his head in the custom of the Near East and fell upon the ground and worshiped. "Naked I came from my mother's womb, and naked I shall return; the Lord gave, and the Lord has taken away; blessed be the name of the Lord" (1:21).

Satan had lost. Job's words of acceptance are so noble that they have become part of our funeral liturgies.

It all might have ended there had not God "rubbed it in" to Satan. "Have you considered my servant Job, that there is none like him on the earth, a blameless and upright man, who fears God and turns away from evil? He still holds fast his integrity, although you moved me against him, to destroy him without cause" (2:3–4).

Without cause. All through the poetic section Job and his counselors search for a cause, a reason for Job's suffering. The quest was doomed from the start. There was no cause. But how does a human being, whose mind relies on a cause-and-effect basis for a sense of meaning, live with *no cause?* Viktor Frankl's *Logotherapy* is based on the assertion that human beings need meaning in life to survive. The book of Job answers this question—but not until the theophany.

Satan is not without a response. He reminded God that God had set limits to Satan's destructive powers: Satan was not to touch Job himself. So let's take away that limit. "Skin for skin! All that a man has he will give for his life. But put forth thy hand now, and touch his bone and his flesh, and he will curse thee to thy face" (2:4–5). Afflict his body! Once more God went along with the challenge—but he still set a limit. "Behold, he (Job) is in your power; only spare his life" (2:6).

So Job is afflicted with "loathsome sores from the sole of his foot to the crown of his head" (2:7). He was so miserable with this affliction that he scraped himself with pieces of pottery to get some relief. The loathsome sores were also loathsome to look upon. This was the last straw for Job's wife, who had endured with him all the other losses. "Do you still hold fast your integrity?" she flaunted in her despair. "Curse God and die" (2:9). Throw in the towel!

But Job "hung in there." "You speak as one of the foolish women would speak." Note that he does not say *she* is a foolish woman. " 'Shall we receive good at the hand of God, and shall we not receive evil?' In all this Job did not sin with his lips" (2:10).

With his lips! Since the prologue made much of Job's concern that his children may have sinned *in their heart,* this description is significant. For it is precisely Job's lips that change when we enter the poetic section. There the simple prior logic of "Shall we receive good and not evil?" gives way to something other.

This contrast between the *lips* of Job in the prologue and in the poetic section has led to various theories about the authorship of the book, as well as the author's motivations. Was the prologue-epilogue written first, and did a psalmist-like person see the need for a deeper dimension to human expression in suffering? Or was the poetic section first, and did a more orthodox person see the need for an orthodox prologue and epilogue?

We need not be locked into such options to account for the difference. If we look at the content of the prologue and poetic section from a theological point of view, another and less radical option is evident. It is not uncommon for people in our culture also who have a great reputation for being outstanding models of piety and reverence, to give the accepted pious and reverent responses to their calamities. Since one of these responses of Job is directed to his wife, it is even more expected that the strong and devout husband would not give expression to his own despair in that moment, but would rather "be strong" for his wife, who was considered more of a dependent than today.

But what was going on in Job's *heart* may have been different, or at least more ambiguous than his verbal statements, and this difference may account for the difference in Job's poetic speeches. Something occurred after Job's philo-

20

sophical words to his wife: the coming of three apparently compassionate friends.

2. The Despair of the Heart

Like Job, the three friends, Eliphaz, Bildad, and Zophar, were men of the East. They had heard of his calamities and "made an appointment together to come to condole with him and comfort him" (2:11). How better to describe a caregiving motivation? When they saw him, however, "they did not recognize him," for his sufferings had taken their toll on his physical appearance. They did not speak—words were obviously inadequate—and instead they wept. Their tears and their other non-verbal symbols or rituals of compassion and grief were more potent than words. "They rent their robes and sprinkled dust upon their heads toward heaven. And they sat with him on the ground seven days and seven nights" in silence, "for they saw that his suffering was very great" (2:12–13).

Those familiar with the present-day customs in the countryside of the East assure us that the seven days and nights can be taken literally. Such an eloquent display of compassion over a prolonged period of time had its effect on Job. Although he remained silent during this time, he was aware of their presence. Could these caring, empathic friends who are giving so generously of their presence understand what was going on in his heart? The hope that they could was the encouragement that Job needed to break this silence and put words to his feelings. His despair had caught up with him and was communicated in his silence. The initial reaction to his traumas had passed, and the deeper strains of this reaction were coming to the surface.

So Job opened his mouth, and his lips were no longer the accepting and submissive lips of the prologue. This time his words did not bless the Lord, but neither did they curse the Lord as Satan had predicted and Job's wife had bidden. Rather, Job cursed the day of his *birth* (3:3).

Why, Job laments, should life be given to the "bitter in

soul?" Why can it not all cease with death so that the misery can come to an end? (3:20). Ironically, the one limitation that God had placed on Satan's destructive power now proves to be an unwanted limit for Job. He wants to die from his calamities, and yet he continues to live!

Job's question *why* is more than a question. It is also a protest. As a question, it is associated with guilt. What have I done to deserve all this? Is God punishing me for something? As a protest, it expresses anger, even outrage. Why is God picking on me? What kind of a God would do such a thing? There is no justice, let alone mercy. In fact, whatever justice one may perceive in the universe is a reversal—a perversion—of justice.

The Jobian *why* is a common reaction of sufferers to their suffering, losses, setbacks, and disappointments. I have a friend who grew up in a pious farm family who believed very strongly that God would bless their endeavors if they worked hard and trusted in him. There were years when this belief was tested. But if there was an occasional bad year, it was followed by several good years. But then came successive years of dought. Year followed year of crop failure. The financial crisis created a spiritual crisis. What had gone wrong?

"Why," Job asks, "did I not die at birth, come forth from the womb and expire?" (3:11). All the good days were not worth the agony Job is now in. The very fact that Job had been so prosperous, with so little negativity "within the hedge," now makes the contrast all the more unbearable. Job had no prior experience with deprivation to draw upon. He felt betrayed by life—by God. His good times were all an illusion. One misses something far more after having had it, than if one had never had it. Job is lost—and there are no signposts that he has been this way before. His many losses are threatening to bring on another—the loss of his faith. What kind of a God is God to allow these things to happen to me?

Job's doubt is not about God's existence, but about God's character. Job seems to share the attitude of the psalmist—it is a *fool* who "says in his heart, 'There is no God' " (Ps.

14:1). The word for "fool" in this psalm is the masculine form of the one for "foolish women" to whom Job had disapprovingly referred. Is this a cultural expectation of this age—to doubt God's character rather than God's existence when one's faith is shaken? Perhaps more so than now. However, this is precisely the kind of doubt that C. S. Lewis expresses in *A Grief Observed* as he grieved over the death of his wife. "Not that I am (I think) in much danger of ceasing to believe in God. The real danger is of coming to believe such dreadful things about Him. The conclusion I dread is not 'So there's no God after all,' but 'So this is what God's really like. Deceive yourself no longer.'" C. S. Lewis, *A Grief Observed*, Greenwich, CT.: Seabury Press, 1963, pp. 9–10).

All sufferers recognize their own anguish in the cries of Job against the injustices of the universe. His agony is commensurate with his calamities. Some of us may even feel guilty that at times we can think like Job even without the ostensibly heavy load of Job's catastrophes. Others may feel like Job because they have been hit by successive losses. The Jobian protest—why?—is our natural reaction when the structures and beliefs we had counted on appear to fail us.

Spiritual counselors are wise to assume a Jobian protest within the hearts of the sufferers to whom they minister. Even though the sufferer's lips sound like those of Job in the prologue, they may have their shadow sides of doubt, resentment, and despair, like Job in the poetic section. Being aware of this possibility, however, does not mean that the counselor should probe for it. People—particularly sufferers—have a sixth sense about how much of reality they can tolerate. It is not up to the counselor to push them beyond these limits, for that would be invading their space. But being open to the possibility sharpens the counselor's ears so that they are more likely to hear the clues to the darker side should they be given, and to follow them.

For example, if afflicted counselees assure the spiritual counselor that their faith in God has given them peace in the midst of their pain, the spiritual counselor need not doubt this simply because there may be a shadow side to this assurance. In fact, counselors may want to reflect the sufferer's statement of faith to reinforce it. Yet our professions of faith often carry within them an ambiguity. The very nature of faith implies a tension with doubt; otherwise we would not label it *faith*.

But if people should drop an aside to their words of faith— "but of course there are times"—and then let their voice trail off, the counselor can draw them out:

"Times when you wonder?"

"Yeah—maybe it's all futile," says the sufferer.

"When God seems far away?" the counselor responds.

"That's it," says the sufferer, "and I have discovered that I feel most removed from God when the pain is at its worst."

"What do you do then?" asks the counselor.

"Oh—I have learned just to let myself go," says the sufferer, "like a child would when he is in pain. Then afterward when I feel better I see it differently. God is still with me— and God understands."

"Even when you are doubting God?" asks the counselor.

"Especially then," the sufferer replies. "And I find this very comforting and reassuring."

This sufferer had worked through some darker periods and could accept and live with the shadow side. Yet it strengthened his adaptation to the ambiguity in faith when the sufferer described it to the counselor—something he likely would not have done if the counselor had not heard the clue and drawn him out on how he dealt with the darker times. The sufferer will also feel encouraged to express negative feelings to the counselor in the future.

Our shadow side is accepted by God, but we may at times question his acceptance. Being able to express to a spiritual counselor these doubts and the despair that may go with them, gives the counselor the opportunity to accept them. Through this human bridge, the acceptance of God may be received when it is most needed. As the symbol bearer of the faith, pastors and other Christian counselors are to some extent an incarnation of this faith.

Chapter Two

When the Darkness Threatens the Light

Eliphaz is the first to respond to Job when he finishes his lament. He was, therefore, probably the oldest of these three friends and the most learned. The comparison of their speeches would substantiate the latter. But despite his learning, his response is emotional. He is shocked. Obviously he had not expected this expression of despair from Job. The silent Job with the great reputation for godliness would be expected to break his silence with prologue-like attestations to his faith.

We ought not be overly judgmental of Eliphaz or his friends. What spiritual counselor would not be made uneasy— if not completely thrown off balance—by such despairing words from a sufferer, from whom one had anticipated the opposite? How often have we heard, or expressed *ourselves,* the testimony of spiritual counselors about their ministry to specific saints in their affliction, "I received more from them than I gave. They actually ministered to *me.*"

But one could hardly say that about Job. Uncomfortable with Job's lament, Eliphaz attempted, perhaps compulsively, to silence him. He is more gentle at first in his attempt than in his later speeches; yet his emotional discomfort already shows signs of becoming anger. The feelings he felt *for* Job during the silent period had turned to feelings *against* him— from feeling *with* to feeling *threatened.* Thus ended his compassion.

Even Eliphaz' offer to respect Job's space is quickly retracted. "If one ventures a word with you, will you be offended? Yet who can keep from speaking?" (4:2). While he wants to be polite, Job's words have demanded a rebuke.

Eliphaz'*speaking* could be summed up as, "Job, I'm troubled by the way you talk. Dear friend, why can you not practice what you yourself have counseled?" "Your words have upheld him who was stumbling . . . But now it has come to you, and you are impatient; it touches you, and you are dismayed" (5:3–5). Eliphaz was referring to Job's having sat in the gate as an elder and counselor. This reminder of his past role as a counselor is supposed to make him feel guilty over his lamenting and move him to speak more like a counselor should.

1. Reaction to Inner Chaos

It can be frightening to perceive another's inner chaos. It may take courage, even for a counselor, to receive it, acknowledge it verbally, and accept it. This is one reason why the question is often asked about a person who has suffered loss, "How is he/she taking it?" The question may be asked as much for the questioner's sake as for the bereaved. We are much more willing to visit one who is "taking it well" than one who is not. We all have our latent inner chaos and sometimes it emerges out of its latency. This is what we perhaps fear in witnessing the chaos of another. We all also have our limits; witnessing a friend's inner chaos may be more than we can take. The verbal expression of this chaos may threaten to arouse our own inner chaos. To protect ourselves, we may avoid the involvement. Pastors, of course, have difficulty avoiding these challenges by staying away personally. All spiritual counselors may, however, avoid them by staying away from them in their conversation. There are many ways we have learned to stay in control of a conversation so that it does not unduly threaten us.

The key issue is whether we have our source of security *within* the emerging chaos, or whether the emerging chaos removes us from our source of security. If the latter were the case, our security would be based on a sense of order. It soon became quite clear that the security of the three friends was rigidly fixed to their own sense of order. This can be seen, for example, in Eliphaz' appeal to Job, "Is not your fear of God your confidence, and the integrity of your ways your hope?" (4:6). This may be an honest appeal. Or it may be a rhetorical question to bring Job to silence through guilt.

Much of what Eliphaz has to say to Job, Job undoubtedly already knew, since they most likely shared the same religious tradition. Yet it no longer spoke to Job. This even includes Eliphaz' wise assurance, repeated elsewhere in both Testaments: "Behold, happy is the man whom God reproves; therefore despise not the chastening of the Almighty. For he wounds, but he binds up; he smites, but his hands heal" (5:17–18; cf. Prov. 3:11–12; Heb. 12:5–6; Rev. 3:19). In these words Eliphaz acknowledges that God is the wounder, which would appeal to Job, but he also says that God's wounding is a rebuke, which Job would not appreciate.

The main deficiency in Eliphaz' argument is that he ignored the protest of Job's *why.* By permitting Job's cursing the day of his birth to turn off his compassion, Eliphaz lost his most valuable resource for counseling Job. He no longer had the bridge to reach Job, and the gulf between them grew.

We have a need, even as spiritual counselors, to supply an answer—to bring order to the chaos—to stay in control. Is this need culturally conditioned? While we should be aware of the differences between the Eastern and Western worlds, and between our day and the era of Job, the three counselors seem also to have this same need. This is but one indication of the way the Book of Job transcends both cultures and ages, and why it has such universal appeal and relevance.

When Eliphaz said, "Think now, who that was innocent ever perished? Or where were the upright cut off?" (4:7), he revealed the frame of reference from which he was operating. If the upright one is not cut off, and Job is upright, all this suffering is temporary, and Job will be healed and restored. But if Job is cut off, then obviously Job is not upright. Eliphaz held out the hope in the beginning that Job was upright. But as the dialogues progress he and his friends became convinced that Job was *not* upright. The goal then is to bring him to repentance.

2. An Appeal for Sympathy

Job appears hurt by Eliphaz' lack of compassion. His initial reaction, however, is to weep rather than become angry. "O that my vexation were weighed, and all my calamity laid in the balances! For then it would be heavier than the sand of the sea; therefore my words have been rash" (6:2–3). Job pleaded for understanding. "Eliphaz, if you only knew the weight I'm carrying, you would understand my rash speaking." One does not normally speak rationally when in excruciating pain. Job says in effect, "You have judged my words without being concerned about what moved me to say them." "Does the wild ass bray when he has grass, or the ox low over his fodder?" (6:5). Job is like a starving animal—desperate—needing relief from the agony of his deprivations.

In appealing to Eliphaz' pity, Job showed how defeated he really felt. In getting no sympathy from others, he lapses into self-pity. The pattern is familiar. Job's complaint over his lot annoys his "comforters" who then proceed to admonish him to see things more positively. The rebuke of the "comforters" is then taken by the sufferer as rejection, and he then whines all the more. But whining and self-pity are even more repulsive to the "comforters" than the previous lamenting, and more censure ensues.

"Is my strength the strength of stones, or is my flesh bronze?" (6:12). How much does God think he can take? He is utterly defeated. "In truth I have no help in me, and any resource is driven from me" (6:13). Job has hit bottom. All sense of self-sufficiency is gone. This is the bottom to which one may need to descend in order to build a firmer foundation for coming back.

Precisely at this point Job's mood changes, and he lashes back at Eliphaz. Why the change? Job's purpose in his appeal to Eliphaz was to regain his compassion. Did he perceive at this point that there was no change forthcoming? If we visualize this exchange, we might now view Eliphaz' countenance as Job pleads and see no change, or perhaps see even more rejection. Job wanted someone to put his arms around him as he described how heavy was his lot, but no arms were proffered. He had gone down as far as he could go—and now anger became his way back.

3. Job Takes to the Offensive

"He who withholds kindness from a friend forsakes the fear of the Almighty" (6:14). This is one of those pivotal verses that is uncertain in its translation. The first part of the sentence is relatively clear: friends should show kindness to one in despair. The Hebrew of the second part is more difficult. Who forsakes the Almighty—the despairing one, or the friend who does not show kindness? The RSV chooses the latter. The value in this choice is that it fits well with what proceeds and follows. It was Eliphaz who implied that Job may have forsaken the fear of the Almighty (4:6). The RSV translation of 6:14 could be Job's response to that insinuation. There is no evidence elsewhere that Job ever thought of himself as forsaking the fear of the Almighty. Rather, Job feels God has forsaken him. This translation also fits well with Job's attack on Eliphaz and his friends that follows through the remainder of the poetic section. Job says it is *Eliphaz* who has forsaken the fear of the Almighty!

Having taken to the offensive against the one who has withheld the compassion (kindness) for which he had pleaded, Job's attack is scathing. His comforters are frauds. "My brethren are treacherous as a torrent-bed, as freshets that pass away" (6:15). They are fair-weather friends. "Dark with ice . . . in time of heat they disappear"(6:16–17). They were a promising oasis in the desert of his despair. Like caravans in the desert he turned toward them to assuage his thirst, but like those same caravans he found himself confronted with a mirage. "The caravans turn aside from their course; they go up into the waste, and perish. The caravans of Tema look, the travelers of Sheba hope. They are disappointed because they were confident; they come thither and are confounded" (6:18–20). This is a powerful metaphor to describe extreme disappointment and disillusion.

4. Counselee's Analysis of the Counselor

Eliphaz had failed as a counselor and Job knows why. "You see my calamity, and are afraid" (6:21). Like many of us, Eliphaz was tense and uneasy in the presence of one who experienced great tragedy. He could control this uneasiness as long as Job was silent, but not after Job had opened his mouth. Then his concern was for his own needs, rather than for Job's, and his speech was a defense of his own anxiety. Instead of functioning as a physician of the soul, he became a defender of his own view of God and of God's justice in the world. As a physician, one is concerned with the hurt—how it can be cared for and healed. But for Eliphaz, Job's expression of his hurt was a threat to Eliphaz' own interpretation of life.

When the needs of the other are the center of our attention, we *respond* in empathy. We move *toward* the other. On the other hand, when we are threatened by the other's needs, we *react*. We move *away* from the other. In responding, the caregiver in us comes forth and we are drawn out of ourselves in compassionate identification with the other. In reacting, our defensiveness takes over and we become preoccupied with our own tension and discomfort.

Instead of understanding Job's rashness, that is, the emotional nature of Job's despair, Eliphaz held him to a rational account of his words. Job the sufferer sees the incongruity in Eliphaz' approach. "Do you think that you can reprove words, when the speech of a despairing man is wind?" (6:26). In his defensiveness Eliphaz had dealt rationally with an emotional outburst. It made no sense to Job—and it makes no sense in Christian counseling. But it is a stupidity that persists and for good reason.

In our modern and Western world we can be as obtuse as Eliphaz in relating sensibly to a sufferer's emotions. The education of our emotions, in contrast to our intellects, is decidely lacking in our educational system. My class in Pastoral Care and Counseling in a theological seminary is for some students the first opportunity in eighteen years of formal education for the education of their emotions. This, of course, can be disconcerting for some because their conception of knowledge is head knowledge. Suddenly they discover that this kind of knowledge is insufficient for this particular course. They could pass a test easily on paper but do poorly, despite this head knowledge, in a clinical setting where heart knowledge is important. In the dynamics of a counseling relationship the education of the emotions is crucial for effective counseling.

The situation is similar to learning all there is to know about the activity of swimming—the various strokes, the movements of the body—so that one could pass a written test about swimming without having been in the water. In the water, knowledge about swimming goes beyond head knowledge, for then emotions emerge which were not aroused on the paper test—fear, even panic. One wants only to get out to the safety of land. There can be a similar panic and a similar desire to exit from a counseling encounter. This is why classes in pastoral care and counseling need to be accompanied by clinical experience under supervision. It is a combination of a classroom and a human relations laboratory, and each is a learning stimulus to the other.

Job's speeches are an illustration of the kind of communication that would demand heart as well as head knowledge. Job would be difficult to listen to for even the most experienced counselor, because his descriptions of his agony exclude the possibility of hope—they are expressions of despair. A good example is the following: "When I say, 'My bed will comfort me, my couch will ease my complaint,' then thou (God) dost scare me with dreams and terrify me with visions, so that I would choose strangling and death rather than my bones (or pains). I loathe my life: I would not live for ever" (7:13–16). Job has no peace even when he sleeps, for then he is tormented with nightmares. He prefers death to the life he is now living. These are hard words to hear, let alone to accept.

If Eliphaz had wanted to intimidate Job into silence, it didn't work. Since death is a final end in Job's thinking, and since he believes he can scarcely live much longer, why should he weigh his words or be temperate in his expression? What does he have to lose? "Therefore I will not restrain my mouth; I will speak in the anguish of my spirit; I will complain in the bitterness of my soul" (7:11). Whether they like to hear what to them are blasphemies or not, if they choose to remain with Job, they will have no choice but to hear.

Since Eliphaz has implied that Job's sin is the cause of his suffering, Job demands to know directly from God why his transgressions should be important enough to justify inflicting such suffering. "If I sin, what do I do to thee, thou watcher of men? Why hast thou made me thy mark?" (7:20). Why should the sin of a puny human being be so important to God Almighty? Has God nothing better to do than be a "watcher of men?" Job believes he has become a mark—a target—for God's arrows, and he wants to know why—why me! Previously he had referred to these arrows as poisonous: "For the arrows of the Almighty are in me; my spirit drinks of their poison" (6:4).

Job has verbalized his dark side. Often this side of our nature shoots through our consciousness in a rapid in-and-out fashion, so that it may be barely recorded in our memory. The advantage in verbalizing it to another is that it helps to fasten it in our consciousness so that we can cope with the reality of our total person. The disadvantage, as Job discovered, is that others are made uncomfortable by such verbalizing, and in their uneasiness they may seek to stop the verbalizing—either by not responding to it, so the sufferer is discouraged from continuing, or by attempting to counteract it with opposing positives, or, as Eliphaz did, with a rebuke. We all have our dark side, and too often our light side is dependent on keeping the dark side hidden. The light side that is genuine and secure needs to shine *in* the darkness as an assurance that the darkness cannot overcome it.

Chapter Three

The Turned-Off and Shaken Counselor

Enter Bildad, the second counselor. He pounces on Job's admission of rashness. "How long will you say these things, and the words of your mouth be a great wind?" (8:2). Obviously, Job's appeal for understanding had missed its mark; Like Eliphaz, Bildad simply could not respond compassionately to Job's despair. The threat inherent in Job's rashness evoked only rebuke from Bildad.

1. Pressure to Conform

Once in a censuring mood, Bildad let go with a "low blow." In the prologue Job was very concerned about his children. After they feasted together he offered sacrifices for them, lest they had "sinned, and cursed God in their hearts" (1:5). Now these children are dead. In defense of the justice operative in the universe, Bildad rubbed Job's sensitive spot. "If your children have sinned against him (God), he has delivered them into the power of their transgression" (8:4). Wasn't their behavior responsible for their tragic deaths?

Based on this cause-and-effect principle, Bildad offered Job a solution to his dilemma. "If you will seek God and make supplication to the Almighty, if you are pure and upright, surely then he will rouse himself for you and reward you with a rightful habitation" (8:5–6). Though Bildad's solution is simplistic, he fortifies it with an appeal to tradition. "For inquire, I pray you, of bygone ages, and consider what the fathers have found; . . . Will they not teach you, and tell you, and utter words out of their understanding?" (8:8,10).

Bildad concluded on a coercive note. "Papyrus cannot grow where there is no marsh," he warns, "nor can reeds flourish where there is no water. Such is the plight of those who show by the path they have taken that they have forgotten God" (8:11–13). But there is a promise to those who conform—or is it a bribe? "He (God) will fill your mouth with laughter, and your lips with shouting" (8:21).

2. A Defiant Resistance

Job's initial response to Bildad is frustration. "Truly I know that it is so." Though Job still has respect for tradition, this very tradition has him in a bind. "But how can a man be just before God? If one wished to contend with him, one could not answer him once in a thousand times" (9:2–3). It's a hopeless predicament—how can a mortal man dispute with God? "Though I am innocent, I cannot answer him (God); I must appeal for mercy to my accuser" (9:15). The contest is futile. "Though I am innocent, my own mouth would condemn me; though I am blameless, he would prove me perverse" (9:20).

Futile or not, Job persists. For Job to admit guilt would have been to surrender his honesty, since he knew he had lived by faith. At the expense of his own security, he can admit only to an irrational guilt. He feels doomed to judgment, not because he is aware of any transgressions that would account for his plight, but only because his God is capricious in his transcendence. This kind of guilt, however, puts no meaning into life, for it is guilt that cannot be removed, since it denies God's grace toward those who are faithful. Job feels no responsibility for this kind of guilt; rather he feels trapped by it. There is no pattern of consistency that he can follow. Whether he is innocent or guilty, his judgment is the same.

To Bildad's rhetorical question, "Does God pervert justice?" (8:3), Job reacts with a defiant *yes!* "The earth is given into the hands of the wicked; he (God) covers the face of its judges" (9:24). Does Bildad resent this charge? Then let him come up with an alternative. "If it is not he (God), who then is it?" (9:24).

This is a good question, a question that spiritual counselors need the courage to face. Rabbi Harold Kushner faced it in *When Bad Things Happen to Good People,* and concluded that God is not omnipotent; many things are beyond his control. Christians have read this book in phenomenal numbers. Does God will human catastrophe? If so, why? If not, who is accountable? Can God prevent them? If so, why does he not always do so? If not, is God helpless against the forces of evil?

The frank facing of these questions helps the sufferer to resolve them. Sufferers may differ, however, on how they resolve them. Spiritual counselors do not need to have answers before they can deal with the questions.

As a sufferer, Job blames God for his pains. "For he (God) crushed me with a tempest, and multiplies my wounds without cause" (9:17).

3. Desire for a Mediator

In his frustration over getting no word from God, Job longs for a go-between, an umpire, a mediator. This is an important theme in the book and in the forthcoming dialogues, and continues to differentiate Job's religious perspective from that of his counselors. The gulf between humans and God is so infinite that Job's only hope for contact is for some sort of mediator. "There is no umpire between us, who might lay his hand upon us both" (9:33). If there were such a mediator, Job could take his case before him. The inherent dread of any confrontation with the Almighty terrifies Job (9:34). If God wants to be fair, let him remove this dread. "Let him take his rod away from me, and let not dread of him terrify me. Then I would speak without fear of him, for I am not so in myself" (9:34–35).

By putting words to this dread, Job seems to have released its hold over him. Since he "loathed his life" anyway, why should he not "give free utterance to his complaint?" (10:1). Believing he has nothing to lose, Job unleashed his attack directly to God. "Does it seem good to thee to oppress, to despise the work of thy hands and favor the designs of the wicked?" (10:3) . . . "Thy hands fashioned and made me; and now thou dost turn about and destroy me" (10:8).

Job's search for meaning in his suffering seems futile. "If I am wicked, woe to me! If I am righteous, I cannot lift up my head, for I am filled with disgrace and look upon my affliction. And if I lift myself up, thou dost hunt me like a lion, and again work wonders against me; thou dost renew thy witnesses against me, and increase thy vexation toward me; thou dost bring fresh hosts against me" (10:15–17).

After this expression of being trapped by God, Job again lamented the day of his birth. "Why didst thou bring me forth from the womb? Would that I had died before any eye had seen me, and were carried as though I had not been, carried from the womb to the grave" (10:18–19). Any hope for recovery is also futile. All Job wants now is for God to "let him alone" for the little time he has left, so that he can have a little comfort—a little peace—before he dies. "Are not the days of my life few? Let me alone that I may find a little comfort before I go whence I shall not return, to the land of gloom and deep darkness, the land of gloom and chaos, where light is as darkness" (10:20–22). At this point, death for Job is only a hope for the end of his miserable life, and not a hope for a resurrection to a better life.

4. From Condoling to Shaming

If Eliphaz was shocked to hear Job curse the day of his birth, how will Zophar, the third counselor, react to Job cursing it directly to God? Whatever hope Job had of evoking compassion from his comforters was shattered by Zophar's reply: "When you mock, shall no one shame you?" (11:3). The counselors have changed from their original goal of condoling with Job and comforting him because of his pain, to shaming him because of his "mockery." Obviously, their initial compassion has become a casualty of the increasingly strident dialogues. If Job persists unchallenged, however, he will shake the foundation of his counselors' security and conception of God. Hence Zophar's need to stop him. His anger may well be his defensive reaction to his own anxiety. Job has become a threat. Consequently, Zophar interprets Job's "letting it all hang out" as mockery of God rather than therapy.

In his anger, Zophar flails wildly at his "opponent." "Know then that God exacts of you less than your guilt deserves" (11:6). Anyone who talks as Job—who "mocks" without "shame"—is simply not a righteous person. He is fortunate that God allows him still to live, let alone to talk. In fact, Zophar seems to long for such retaliation. "But oh, that God would speak, and open his lips to you" (11:5). Since Job continued unrestrained by any act of God against him, the three counselors continue shaken and defensive. The vehemence of Zophar's attack indicates the degree to which he as well as the others had been affected by Job's attack of their theological and philosophical system.

5. Counselees who Shake Counselors

Not all counselees respond as we counselors hope, and the degree to which they differ from our expectations may affect us emotionally. Christian counseling is a dialogical ministry. This means we cannot predict or control what will happen in the counseling session.

This lack of predictability differentiates Christian counseling from other forms of ministry, such as preaching and even teaching. If we prepare a sermon, we can with great probability predict what we will say throughout the sermon. Not so with Christian counseling. It is good to have plans (they are included in verbatim writeups of counseling sessions), but these plans may have to be set aside, depending on the agenda which the counselee brings to the session.

Things can seem to get out of control when the counselee reacts in unanticipated or highly emotional ways—as Job did. This can create apprehension within the counselor, and like Job's counselors, we may try to regain control. The more resistive the counselee is to our control, the more coercive we may become.

I myself become aware of my negative reaction toward a

counselee through the heaviness I feel as I approach the next counseling session. When I ask myself what it is that is dampening my feelings, on each occasion I come up with the same answer. This individual, couple, or family has not been responding to the counseling as I had hoped. The heaviness is due to my anticipation of another no-progress session or even a reversal of progress. Obviously, I am reluctant to endure the frustration this person is going to generate. I may sense in this counselee a resistance to change—or a habituation to regressive ways—that I feel inadequate to overcome. Should I share with them my heaviness or would this simply add more pressure to someone who does not deal well with pressure?

What I see going on within me is an unwillingness to accept the process by which most progress is made in counseling, namely, that regression is often a natural followup to a forward movement, and resisting this pattern may only prolong the regression. When I accept the situation as it is, I am often surprised in the opposite direction, namely, that progress often follows regression.

Counselees who do not respond as we counselors anticipate are at first intimidating to us. Usually when we are intimidated we try harder to please in an attempt to justify ourselves as competent to the counselee. If this attempt to please should fail, however, we may become even more defensive. Our uneasiness and anxiousness about the conversation turn into irritation and annoyance toward the counselee. Our need then is to set the counselee straight. In an attempt to end the annoyance, the discomfited counselor may become more argumentative than dialogical. Using combative tactics under the guise of superior reasoning, the counselor now is trying to "shame the mocker."

Pastoral and other Christian counselors may think that other professional counselors, before whom we tend to feel inferior, would be too professional or secure to allow themselves to be shaken by their clients. Psychoanalyst Ann Miller says otherwise. A question she says she is frequently asked when speaking to fellow psychoanalysts is how to deal with the "undesirable feelings" some patients arouse within them. Miller says she avoids answering the question, believing they should discuss this matter among themselves to shed light on the intra and inter-personal dynamics behind the question.

Miller views her own feelings of irritation and annoyance at specific patients as part of the communication process. "I always assume that the patient has no other way of telling me his story than the one he actually uses. Seen thus, all feelings arising in me, including irritation, belong to his coded language and are of great heuristic value"(Ann Miller, *Prisoners of Childhood*, New York: Basic Books, 1981, p.77). For Miller, the analyst's emotional reaction to the patient's communication constitutes an extension of that communication.

Miller's interpretation of the psychoanalyst's reaction to the patient may be helpful also to spiritual counselors. If one at least raises the question in his/her own mind when feeling emotional discomfort—"Is what is going on within me needed for my reception of what the counselee is desiring to communicate?"—this momentary reflection may influence one to respond in ways that enhance rather than frustrate the communication process.

6. Accepting Our Limits

We all have our limits of toleration. It is important to realize and accept them. The acceptance of our own limits will help us focus on what is happening in the dialogue more than if we become defensive. Otherwise, we will be hindered in coping realistically with our emotional reactions to frustrating counselees. Our theology of God's grace in Christ gives us permission to be limited. As Christian counselors, we are under no mandate always to be adequate to the task. Counselees who disturb us do so usually because we sense we are failing them. When we realize we do not have to succeed in order to be justified, we can tolerate our failures. Then the counselee becomes less of a threat and more of a person in our eyes, and as a result our counseling may improve.

Our emotional reaction to frustrating counselees, however, can overwhelm even our awareness of our theology of God's grace in Christ. Like Job's three counselors, our efforts then can become counterproductive to the counseling dialogue. Counselors, even veteran counselors, need a supervisor—a colleague from whom they can receive feedback on their counseling. Such supervision is a requirement not only for membership in the American Association of Pastoral Counselors, but also for continuing as a member. A professional outside the counseling relationship needs to evaluate the emotional conflict that has been developing. We may discover that simply sharing the situation with our chosen supervisor is sufficient for us to see more clearly what is happening in the relationship with the counselee. Or perhaps the problem has become so specifically our own that we need counseling ourselves from our supervisor to free ourselves from our negative reactions. With this support we may be able to see that our emotional reaction was really an extension of the counselee's communication. Then we are able once again to take on the responsibilities of a counselor.

Chapter Four

Living with
Unanswered
Questions

Zophar's attack brings a sarcastic counterattack from Job. "No doubt you are the people, and wisdom will die with you" (12:2). The points upon which they are hammering—who does not know them? They are the well-worn religious dogmas in which all of them were reared. He will not let them talk down to him. "I am not inferior to you. Who does not know such things as these?" (12:3).

1. Finding Strength Through Anger

We witness in this interchange anger's integrating effect on Job. While he often sinks into depression, his comforters so rile him that he bounces back in anger. A coach may deliberately rile his phlegmatic team to motivate them to do their best. Some counselors do the same with their apathetic counselees, although this is not my style as a pastoral counselor. I have, however, evoked anger from counselees without intending to do so. In every such instance that I can recall, the anger seemed to be a strengthening influence. When a counselee expresses anger toward the counselor, either verbally or non-verbally, it is important that the counselor both acknowledge and accept this anger.

Job believes his calamities have made him a "laughingstock" to his friends. For a man of his prestige to be laughed at is a reversal of justice. "I, who called upon God and he answered me, a just and blameless man, am a laughingstock" (12:4). Why would anyone—let alone one's friends—make a sufferer the butt of jokes?

Job believes he knows why. "In the thought of one who is at ease there is contempt for misfortune; it is ready for those whose feet slip" (12:5). Is there a tendency for those who are *up* to kick those who are *down?* Is there no built-in compassion for those "whose feet slip"? Marie Antonette's callous dismissal of the poor of Paris who had no bread—"Let them eat cake!"—is a gross example of a common tendency. "Let them behave themselves, or live right, or work at it!" We tend not to allow ourselves to *feel* with them in their pain. Pain hurts, even the pain of compassion. If we are to feel good about our good fortune, we need to judge those with bad fortune for "bringing it on themselves."

But to Job it is really *God* who is unfair. "The tents of robbers are at peace, and those who provoke God are secure, who bring their god in their hand" (12:6). In contrast, the "just and blameless" do the suffering!

2. Questioning the Traditional Answers

Since his comforters are where he himself used to be in thinking and believing, their words are judged by Job's ears as stale—like stale food to the tongue (12:11). Rather than argue with Zophar's insistence on the sovereignty of God, Job takes to the offensive by asking who would doubt this sovereignty. Even the plant and animal kingdoms acknowledge it (12:7–9). *Of course* it is the hand of God that has afflicted him. But this knowledge only aggravates Job's anguish by forcing him to question what he previously would not have questioned—that God was gracious toward him. New situations bring forth new questions and, hopefully, new answers. However, the time lag between the raising of the questions and their resolution can be agonizing. Perhaps this is why Rainer Maria Rilke advised a young poet to "be patient toward all that is unsolved in your heart," and to "try to love the questions themselves" (Henri Nouwen, *Reaching Out*, Harper, 1975, p.28).

Job is no longer innocent—his eyes have been opened—and he is rebelling against the Job who used to be. The answers are simple when one does not have the problem. Those who have the problem raise questions that their previous frame of reference did not encompass.

Mark had been reared in a Christian home in which it was implicitly believed that God would protect the faithful from calamities. And it seemed to work that way in his family. But when Mark's fiancee was killed by a drunken driver, not only Mark but also his faith was devastated.

"I don't know what I believe anymore," he told his pastor.

"Because of what happened?" his pastor asked.

"Yes—it's knocked the props out from under my faith."

"You feel betrayed?"

"Well—yes, I guess I do."

"It shouldn't have happened," said the pastor.

"No," Mark said, frowning deeply. "I believed God led her to me so that we might be married."

"And look what happened."

"And by a drunken driver! What chance did she have? It's not right." He was moved to tears.

"It seems unfair—unjust, doesn't it," the pastor said.

"Right," Mark said, showing appreciation for being understood. "So how do I live with that?"

Obviously Mark's previous faith could not encompass a tragedy like his fiancee's senseless death. The faith that comes to him now will be a faith that *can*.

What can spiritual counselors offer to such questions? Their offering reflects what God offers—not simple answers to the Jobian *why*, but a sustaining relationship in which the questioners can work out or at least approach answers they can live with. In this ministry the Christian caregivers represent the solidarity of the congregation which is upholding the sufferer by its compassion and prayers in Jesus' name.

Job grew weary of arguing with those who did not have the basis in experience for understanding his predicament. "Worthless physicians are you all" (13:4). All they do is "whitewash with lies" (13:4). He longs for those seven days and nights when they communicated through silence. "Oh that you would be silent, and it would be your wisdom!" (13:5).

Job's attack on his counselors reveals an ambivalence in his denial of God's justice. After accusing them of taking God's side in the conflict, of defending God at the expense of facing reality, denying his justification and righteousness through faith, Job warned them that this would bring God's ire upon them. "Will you speak falsely for God, and speak deceitfully for him? Will you show partiality toward him, will you plead the case for God? Will it be well with you when he seeks you out? Or can you deceive him, as one deceives a man? He will surely rebuke you if in secret you show partiality" (13:7–10).

God neither needs nor wants spiritual counselors to defend God. Since the three counselors have disqualified themselves by their partiality toward God, why should Job listen to them? "Your maxims are proverbs of ashes, and your defenses are defenses of clay" (13:12).

3. Taking His Case to God

Having dispensed with his incompetent counselors, Job turns his attention to God: "I will speak, and let come on me what may" (13:13). Though God may slay him he will not back down— rather, he says, "I will defend my ways to his face" (13:15).

Job may have frightened himself by the sound of his own bravado. Before he can really present his case with such confidence, he makes two requests of God. "Only grant two things to me, then I will not hide myself from thy face: Withdraw thy hand far from me, and let not dread of thee terrify me" (13:20–21). God's transcendence is magnified against Job's finitude, and Job is frightened. We humans are as transitory as a flower. By what logic then does God bring such frail ones to judgment? "Wilt thou frighten a driven leaf and pursue dry chaff?" (13:25). If Job is a sinner, he is a helpless sinner. "Who can bring a clean thing out of an unclean?" (14:4).

In his despair Job sees only the determined side of human existence. Humans are only "hirelings" (14:16). Since God

46

has appointed bounds that humans cannot pass, why does he not then "look away from him and desist"? (14:6)

"Look away from him, and desist." Like other sufferers Job cannot understand why God has singled him out. "Let me alone till I swallow my spittle" (7:19). The thought of God's presence is anything but a comfort. "Wilt thou frighten a driven leaf?" Martin Luther understood Job's negative awareness of God from his own suffering—his *Anfechtung* or despair. He described such a sufferer as wishing that "God were not God, so that he might not suffer such things from him" (Gordon Rupp, *The Righteousness of God,* New York: Philosophical Library, 1953, p.112).

If the present is intolerable, the future for Job is just as bad. Even a tree is better off than humans, for if it is cut down it will sprout again, "But man dies, and is laid low; man breathes his last, and where is he?" (14:10).

But Job cannot leave his future so bleak. "Oh that thou wouldst hide me in Sheol ... that thou wouldst appoint me a set time, and remember me! If a man die, shall he live again? All the days of my service I would wait, till my release should come" (14:13–14). When Job holds to this hope, God becomes his friend. "Thou wouldest call, and I would answer thee; thou wouldest long for the work of thy hands" (14:15).

Job's despair is too deeply embedded to allow his hopes to soar for long. He descends again into desolation. "But the mountain falls and crumbles away ... so thou destroyest the hope of man ... He feels only the pain of his own body, and he mourns only for himself' (14:18–19,22). Pain can turn us in on ourselves, diminishing our capacity for compassion toward others.

4. What Sufferers Really Need

What are a counselor's feelings when a devastated counselee asks the agonizing questions regarding their calamities—questions for which there are no easy or simple answers. In my seminar with doctoral students in pastoral care and counseling, I discussed such a counselee. "What do you say to such a person?" a student asked. Another said with a shudder, "I wouldn't know what to say." Their countenances were saying, "I dread being in these kinds of situations."

I cannot imagine anyone enjoying being in such a situation. But as spiritual counselors we are in them all too frequently. How frustrating it can be when we cannot supply the answer that people so desperately want. Without such answers to these agonizing questions of why, what is the purpose of our counseling and care?

What goes on within us when we find ourselves in this predicament? Is God on trial here? Is the counselor? Do we feel inadequate or even resented in such moments? Pastors are the natural target for peoples' anger when they are struck by calamity and tragedy. They are the symbol-bearers for a system of divine providence. When in peoples' minds this system has gone awry, who is going to take the flack?

What—or who—is the source of the security that enables a counselor to keep the focus on the counselee rather than on the need to justify his own presence and position in such a moment? This security begins as the counselor faces his own doubts regarding this providential system. These doubts may be one reason why counselors can feel the anxiety also in that moment. Although these doubts are anything but comforting, we need to come to terms with them. Rather than aberrations on the system of providence, they are part and parcel with it in this fallen world. The counselee's questions are also the counselor's questions, although at the moment they may be laying quiet rather than being at fever pitch. But they can hardly remain quiet when aroused by the intensity of the counselee's demands.

False assumptions may accompany one's understanding of faith. When I reminded a fellow sufferer that nowhere in our biblical tradition are we led to believe that trusting in God means that one will be spared the calamities of life, she responded, "I suppose I knew that in my head, but I didn't want to know it and so I didn't." Even Jesus' own disciples at first did not want to accept the necessity of his suffering, nor their own suffering as they followed him. It is the sense of betrayal that makes the questions so fiercely penetrating. Like Job, the sufferers feel that justice has been perverted.

When we are at peace with the questions because the questions go with life in this world under the cross, we are in position to give the agonizing Jobs what they need. We can "hang in there" with them as they shout out their laments and point at us with their questions. Both counselor and counselee know there are no answers. But someone needs to hear them out—to respond understandingly even when one senses that one is being attacked. For God is more than an answer. As sufferers receive the support they need in the person of an understanding and compassionate counselor, as they lash out in their hurt and anger, they can come in their own time to know their own peace with God—although their questions remain unanswered.

Chapter Five

The Way Up
May Be Down

Eliphaz' second speech reinforces Zophar's observation. "Your own mouth condemns you, and not I" (15:6). Eliphaz sounds proleptically like another judge of another sufferer. After listening to the prisoner Jesus acknowledge that he was the Christ, the high priest who was judging him said, "Why do we still need witnesses? You have heard his blasphemy" (Mk. 14:62–63).

Eliphaz' speech with its many metaphors and descriptions reasserts the justice of the universe, and could be summed up by 15:20: "The wicked man writhes in pain all his days, through all the years that are laid up for the ruthless."

After Eliphaz finished speaking, Job offered him a good insight. "I also could speak as you do, if you were in my place" (16:4). However, Job might also do things differently. "I could strengthen you with my mouth, and the solace of my lips would assuage your pain" (16:5). By supplying "or" as a correlative conjunction between verses 4 and 5, the contrasting actions become clear: if Job were in their place, he could either accuse them (v. 4) or console them (v. 5).

1. The Brutality of God
But Job's pain continues unassuaged and unabated whether he speaks out or keeps quiet. Nothing helps. "Surely now God has worn me out" (16:6–7). What follows is one of the most devastating accusations of God's brutality in all literature. God has "made desolate all my company . . . shriveled me up . . . torn me in his wrath . . . gnashed his teeth at me . . . casts me into the hands of the wicked . . . broke me asunder . . . seized me by the neck and dashed me to pieces

... set me up as his target ... slashes open my kidneys ... pours out my gall on the ground ... breaks me with breach upon breach ... runs upon me like a warrior" (16:7–14).

The temptation for sufferers is to displace their anger toward God onto others such as pastors, fellow church members, and family members. Job has the courage to be direct—to lash out at God whom he holds responsible for his calamities. After "letting God have it," his confidence in God returns. "O earth, cover not my blood, and let my cry find no resting place. Even now, behold, my witness is in heaven, and he that vouches for me is on high" (16:18–19). This hope for a heavenly witness is another repetition of Job's hope for a mediator.

Job is under no illusion in this brief resurgence of confidence. "My spirit is broken, my days are extinct, the grave is ready for me. Surely there are mockers about me, and my eye dwells on their provocation" (17:1–2). It has happened too often before. Yet Job is ready for the "mockers," and let there be no doubt about who they are. "But you, come on again, all of you, and I shall not find a wise man among you" (17:10).

Whatever hope there is will come in the absence of all hope. "If I look for Sheol as my house, if I spread my couch in darkness, if I say to the pit, 'You are my father,' and to the worm, 'My mother,' or 'My sister,' where then is my hope? Who will see my hope? Will it go down to the bars of Sheol? Shall we descend together into the dust?" (17:13–16). Job sounds like St. Francis of Assisi in reverse. Instead of identifying with other creatures of God as his mother, brother, and sister as Francis did, Job asks if his kinship is with the symbols of death and destruction—the *pit* into which the dead enter and the *worm* that destroys decaying bodies. Nothing tangible in the universe can add anything positive to his miserable situation.

2. Outrage Over Humiliation

Knowing the defensiveness of the counselors we would not expect them to let this charge against God go unrebuked.

Bildad rises to the occasion. "You who tear yourself in your anger, shall the earth be forsaken for you, or the rock be removed from its place?" (18:4). Does the universe have to adjust to you? But Bildad has nothing further to offer and so he rehashes the old theme. "Yea, the light of the wicked is put out, and the flame of his fire does not shine" (18:5).

Job is deeply offended by his counselors for making "my humiliation an argument against me" (19:5). This is the common "Catch-22" for sufferers. Once a person is down, we attempt to account for it by something they have done to "bring it on themselves." This is the "blame the victim" syndrome. We feel better if we can give a rationale for such tragedies. Otherwise our sense of meaning is threatened. To all of this Job cries, "Violence!" We would say, "Foul." "I know," he says, "that God has put me in the wrong, and closed his net about me . . . I call aloud, but there is no justice" (19:5–7). He feels trapped by a sovereign power who has "walled up my way" and "set darkness upon my paths" (19:8). "He has kindled his wrath against me, and counts me as his adversary" (19:11). In Job's eyes a formerly cooperative relationship has turned adversarial.

In describing the "wall" and the "darkness," Job paints a pathetic picture of his social rejection. How humiliating for one who had great prestige to have to beseech a servant, and even then the servant does not answer! How devastating to be so physically afflicted that one is repugnant to one's own wife and brothers! How debasing to an older person in a culture where age equals status to be despised and ridiculed even by *children*! (19:16–18).

Job described his rejection so graphically that he himself is overcome by it. With no pride left he reaches out pathetically for sympathy. "Have pity on me, have pity on me, O you my friends . . . why do you, like God, pursue me?" (19:21–22).

3. The Glorious Vision

"Letting it all hang out," may lead to renewed vision. The way *up* may be *down.* Following his descent to the depths of despair, Job rises to the heights of hope. "Oh that my words were written! O that they were inscribed in a book! O that with an iron pen and lead they were graven in the rock forever!" (19:23–24). He knows from experience that his periods of hope do not last, and so he wants to set this one "in concrete."

So saying, he lets his hopes ascend. "For I know that my Redeemer lives, and at last he will stand upon the earth." The Redeemer-umpire-mediator (Hebrew *go'el*) that Job had asked and hoped for he now *sees*. He *knows* his Redeemer *lives*. "And after my skin has been thus destroyed, then from my flesh I shall see God" (19:25–26). Job is convinced that though something violent may destroy his body, yet in this body he will see God. He—Job— will see for *himself*—*his* eyes shall behold God, not the eyes of another (19:27). The wonderful vision is all but too much for Job. "My heart faints (KJV—reins are consumed) within me" (19:27).

As we read this stirring description of Job's vision, we may also *hear* it in Handel's *Messiah*. This great oratorio captures the emotions as well as the words of Job as his spirit soars with the vision of hope. Christians have identified the Redeemer whom Job envisioned as Jesus the Messiah. Psychoanalyst Carl G. Jung sees in Jesus God's answer to Job. God entered into human life in Jesus of Nazareth, and suffered as Job did. Jesus then is uniquely fitted to be Job's *go'el*. In his sufferings Jesus endured the same agony of rejection as Job. His cry in his anguish on the cross parallels not only Psalm 22 but also Job: "My God, my God, why hast thou forsaken me?" (Matt. 27:46). How can Jesus be the mediator between God and humankind and still be forsaken by God? Actually, it is in the experience of forsakenness that he becomes the mediator. His identification—empathy—with humanity had to encompass the nature of human experience—the Jobian experience—and his identification with God had to reckon with God's wrath. Here was the "expiating self-sacrifice offered up to the wrath of God's dark side," as Jung put it (*Answer to Job*, p. 155).

Evidently Job's soaring spirit and stirring hope was not shared by the three counselors. They were simply too defensive to let themselves hear. So Job warns them. In seeking to blame him for his troubles, the counselors were inviting the judgment of God upon themselves (19:28–29).

4. Dealing With Emotional Fluctuation

Job's emotional ups and downs expressed to his counselors are typical of the sufferer. They need to be received by the counselor within the perspective of the Higher Counselor who is the sustaining influence of the counseling relationship. The counselor's awareness of the presence of God provides him or her with the moment-by-moment context within which to listen to the instability of surging emotions. For the Christian counselor, this presence is the presence of the One who has become incarnate as the Redeemer.

This belief in a Redeemer who himself has endured forsakenness in his life on earth has traditionally been a cognitive and affective support to suffering Christians. C. S. Lewis attempted to comfort his grieving friend by describing Christ's own forsakenness and protest against God's apparent rejection. After having been forsaken by all others as he was condemned to crucifixion, Christ had nothing left but God. And to God, God said, "why hast thou forsaken me?" (*Letters to Malcolm Chiefly on Prayer.* N.Y.: Harcourt, Brace and World, Inc., 1963, p. 43).

Yet the value of Christ's mediation through identification with our pain may not be existentially perceived in the moment of despair. In Lewis' own subsequent grief over the death of his wife, for example, he seemed to find Christ's forsakenness of little comfort. "C reminded me," he wrote in *A Grief Observed*, "that the same thing seems to have happened to Christ: 'Why hast thou forsaken me?' I know. Does that make it easier to understand?" (London: Faber and Faber, 1961, p.9).

But it does help the spiritual counselor by providing a context or mindset within which to accept the counselee's protests. The divine-human encounter as we know it in Christ, the Redeemer, encompasses and transcends our counseling.

Within this perspective not everything depends upon the counseling process. Much has gone on prior to the counseling, and much is going on along with the counseling, and much will go on beyond the counseling. Even the counseling session itself may be something other than what either the counselee or counselor perceives. How God perceives it is beyond the certainty of either counselor or counselee. Consequently, hope may lie beyond what is apparent to either of them. For in the context of the presence of God in counseling, both are challenged to "walk by faith, not by sight" (2 Cor. 5:7).

Interpreting the ups and downs of the counselee's communication within the context of the presence of the One who suffered with us and for us, helps the counselor accept and respond constructively to the frequently chaotic dynamics of sufferers who communicate like Job. All that transpires is within God's empathy. This is the "trancendent system" within which the system of spiritual counselor and counselee functions.

5. Achieving Peace in Turbulence

Although none of us finds it easy to listen to the continuous laments of the depressed, some of us find it more difficult than others. Paul, for example, had been a parish pastor for a decade and had several quarters of clinical pastoral education. Yet he found it almost intolerable to listen for any length of time to someone whose expression of hopelessness and gloom continued despite his counseling efforts. After such an experience Paul was an "emotional wreck." As Lewis admitted to Malcolm, "Your darkness has brought me back my own" (*Letters to Malcolm,* p. 44) Paul knew that this inability was an obstacle to his caring and counseling. So he accepted a clinical assignment in a depression unit of a hospital. During a counseling session with a woman (whom he had previously counseled with much emotional discomfort), Paul had an amazing experience. The woman sounded like Job in his most hopeless moments. As she expressed her gloom, Paul became aware that he was listening for the first time to such expressions without feeling panicky. He was relaxed as he listened. He could emphathize with her pain without taking on her depressive mindset.

After what he deemed was sufficient time for the woman to express herself, Paul asked her to join him as he read Psalm 88 to her. This psalm is an unmitigated expression of lament, but expressed within a milieu of prayer. When he asked her if she could identify with the psalmist, she said she surely could. They discussed the psalmist's feelings as he expressed them in prayer. This opened the way for Paul to suggest that they also put her expression of darkness into prayer. As the session closed, the woman thanked Paul for not "painting a positive picture" as he had previously. Paul realized then that he had done this "painting" in an adversarial manner because he was threatened by her hopeless picture.

Probably the most difficult time for us to listen to depressed thinking is after the counselee is feeling better. It is hard not only for the counselee to experience a regression, but also for the counselee's counselor. Like Job, people in depressed moods can seem to come out of it temporarily. But they may also slip back. Then the hopeless expressions are not only threatening because they are hopeless, but also because they seem to undermine what the counselor had perceived as progress toward recovery.

At these times also it may be helpful to remind ourselves as pastoral counselors that God is still present even though God seems hidden, and that God can use even a regression in the process of healing. Within this perspective, success and failure, progress and regression are all contingent impressions and are subject to the larger perspective of the divine perspective. After all, the Redeemer's experience of dereliction was the prelude to his resurrection.

Chapter Six

Only Integrity Remains

As Zophar begins his second discourse by saying, "I hear censure which insults me" (20:3), he shows the level of communication to which they have all now adapted. The discussion has become a heated argument. As Zophar sees it, Job is resisting an age-old axiom. "Do you not know this from of old, since man was placed upon the earth, that the exulting of the wicked is short, and the joy of the godless but for a moment?" (20:4–5). He continues throughout his second speech to provide metaphor upon metaphor in describing the short-lived prosperity of evildoers. "He swallows down riches and vomits them up again ... The possessions of his house will be carried away, dragged off in the day of God's wrath. This is the wicked man's portion from God, the heritage decreed for him by God" (20:15, 28–29).

1. Where is Justice Now?

Job is quick to react. "Bear with me, and I will speak, and after I have spoken, mock on" (21:3). Since Zophar had previously accused Job of mocking, Job now returns the epithet. If what he had charged previously had troubled them, what he now has to say will appall them. Job then proceeds to paint an entirely contrasting picture of the fortunes of evildoers. "They spend their days in prosperity and in peace they go down to Sheol. They say to God, 'Depart from us! We do not desire the knowledge of thy ways. What is the Almighty, that we should serve him? And what profit do we get if we pray to him?'" (21:13–15). In the prologue, Satan taunted God that Job's righteousness was well rewarded. "Does Job fear God for nought?" (1:9). Now Job is saying that the wicked are well aware that there is no advantage in fearing God. In fact, it pays them *not* to fear God.

Job seeks to plug a possible escape in their argument. "You say, 'God stores up their iniquity for their sons ...' " (21:19). If they don't receive the judgment for their ways, their *children* will. The idea of "visiting the iniquity of the fathers upon the children to the third and fourth generation of those who hate me" (Ex. 20:5) was familiar to their thinking. But Job will have none of it. The postponement of justice to another generation is a denial of justice. "Let him (God) recompense it to themselves, that they may know it. ... for what do they care for their houses after them?" (21:19–21).

This indictment of evildoers in Job's generation sounds an ominous warning to our generation. In the industrialization of our planet, we are polluting it—our soil, water, air, and even the protective atmosphere of our space. But since we are not experiencing the immediate effects of this polluting, we are doing little as a world community to stop it. Since it is future generations that will experience the devastation rather than our own, we choose instead to make our financial profits and enjoy our temporary reprieve. If we were "recompensed" in our own lifetime, we might make the necessary changes to save the planet while there is yet time.

Do the counselors appeal to the wisdom of tradition? Let them come out of the clouds and listen to the pragmatists. "Have you not asked those who travel the roads, and do you not accept their testimony?" These people who travel the roads will tell you that "the wicked man is spared in the day of calamity" (21:29–30). These travelers have been around and they know! The indictment against God stands!

Believing he has demolished his counselors' rational depiction of the order of the universe, Job chides them for their lack of honesty. "How then will you comfort me with empty nothings? There is nothing left of your answer but falsehood" (21:34).

2. Ad Hominem Attacks

This is all too much for Eliphaz. In reaction he unleashes a vicious attack on Job's character. It is an old standby: if you cannot deal with your opponent's argument, then attack his or her person. Job's reputation for righteous living has held the counselors somewhat at bay. But after listening to what seemed to them a blasphemous attack on God, this image of righteousness was badly damaged. So without any other evidence, Eliphaz proceeds to attack Job for his unrighteous way of life. "Is not your wickedness great? There is no end to your iniquities. For you have exacted pledges of your brothers for nothing, and stripped them naked of their clothing. You have given no water for the weary to drink, and you have withheld bread from the hungry . . . You have sent widows away empty, and the arms of the fatherless were crushed" (22:5–7, 9). The wildness of Eliphaz' accusations could indicate how shaky he felt under Job's attack of his system.

What does a counselor do when a counselee attacks their basis for security? Very few of us would let go in counter-attack as did Eliphaz. Yet there are more subtle and "rationally defensible" ways of putting down an intimidating counselee. When they resist our methodology, we may suggest that they are being defensive. Or we can attempt to corner them by dealing logically with their irrational behavior. When counselees become offensive like Job, they leave themselves open to inconsistencies. Counselors may attempt to stay in control—or retain the power— by pointing to inconsistencies as evidence of the weakness in the counselee's offense. If the pressure increases, the counselor may subtly threaten the counselee by warning them of the consequences of their actions. If all else fails, the *pastoral* counselor can imply or even assert that the counselee is judged by the Scriptures. We may even use a few quotations to back up the indictment.

I refer to these procedures as putdowns rather than confrontations because the motivation is an attempt, sometimes desperate, to stay in control. Like Eliphaz, the counselor is on the offensive because he or she is on the defensive. Because the mindset as well as the emotional state is different than when a counselor decides to confront a counselee, the effect is different on the counselee. It is an attack, actually a counter-attack, and is perceived as such. To Zophar's credit, he admitted his ego had been bruised by Job's accusations. He was *insulted*. In contrast, Eliphaz does not acknowledge his feelings but instead cruelly attacks Job's character. While I do not wish to make too much of this differentiation between the counselors (since there is but a pastoral perception to substantiate it), the fact remains that this difference in counselor openness, and consequently, in counseling approaches, is crucial to effective counseling. Counselors who can share their feelings of frustration and anger with their counselees are less likely to engage in battles for control with them than counselors who have a need to simulate this control by concealing those feelings which indicate their sense of control is threatened. They are less likely then to attack the self-esteem of their counselees to put them down.

3. Rejection of Silence

Job's immediate reaction to Eliphaz' attack on his righteousness is to long to talk with God, since it is so futile to continue the argument with his counselors. "Oh, that I knew where I might find him, that I might come even to his seat! I would lay my case before him and fill my mouth with arguments" (23:3–4). Job believes that if he had the opportunity he could convince God of his innocence. But God is nowhere to be found. "Behold, I go forward, but he is not there; and backward, but I cannot perceive him; on the left hand I seek him, but I cannot behold him; I turn to the right hand, but I cannot see him" (23:8–9)

But he is convinced that God sees *him*. Because God "knows the way that I take," Job can with confidence refute the charges Eliphaz has made against his character (23:10–12). At the same time Job is in dread of God, and his heart grows faint (23:15–16). As darkness descends on his spirit, he cries out, "Why are not times of judgment kept by the

Almighty, and why do those who know him never see his days?" (24:1). Why does God not sit in the gate so that people could bring their pleas for justice to him? Why cannot God be like us humans?

After Eliphaz' attack, Job felt rejected by his counselors and turned to his only hope—God. But after affirming his confidence in God, he receives only silence, and ultimately he interprets the silence also as rejection. In his downfall Job identifies with the poor and the afflicted of the earth. They seem to have no advocates—only oppressors. "They thrust the poor off the road" (24:4). "They lie all night naked, without clothing . . . they are wet with the rain of the mountains . . . hungry, they carry the sheaves . . . they tread the wine presses, but suffer thirst . . . the dying groan, and the soul of the wounded cries for help . . . " (24:7, 10, 11, 12). Where is God in all of this oppression, in "man's inhumanity to man?" Job is bitter: in spite of the cries of the afflicted, "God pays no attention to their prayer" (24:12).

In this sense of rejection from his friends and from God, Job turns to the only ones with whom he can identify: the oppressed and downtrodden of the earth. He turns to other victims like himself, for whom no one turns a hand to help. He can find company with them in lamenting an indifferent providence.

4. A Challenge to Integrity

Bildad does not react or respond to Job's charge of divine indifference to human suffering. Instead, he offers doxologies to God's omnipotence. Before such a God no human being can claim to be righteous. If "even the moon is not bright and the stars are not clean in his (God's) sight; how much less man, who is a maggot, and a son of man, who is a worm!" (25:5–6). The implication behind the doxology is—who does Job think he is to charge God as he has!

For those interested in tracing the origins of depicting humanity as a worm—or even as maggot—Bildad is already one of the sources. His need to exalt the divinity leads to a denigration of humanity. The significance of the one demands the insignificance of the other. It is a position consonant with their legalism and worldview, and a position that Job defiantly rejects. His reaction is full of the irony and satire with which he has repeatedly viewed his comforters. "How you have helped him who has no power! . . . How you have counseled him who has no wisdom . . . with whose help have you uttered words, and whose spirit has come forth from you?" (26:2–4).

Yet Bildad touched a raw nerve; Job has known his moment of dread—of terror before the presence of the Almighty. He had even been tempted to surrender his defiance for fear of divine retribution. Yet despite this frightening aspect of carrying on a solitary fight against the injustice of God, Job will not yield. "My lips will not speak falsehood . . . Far be it from me to say you are right; till I die I will not put away my integrity from me" (27:4–5). His heart, he insists, does not reproach him for any of his days (27:6). An overstatement? Of course! It is his offensive defense against the accusations of his counselors.

Job's choice of his integrity over bowing to pressure is a familiar depiction of humanity at its best. The noble spirit values integrity as a virtue that cannot be compromised. Holding fast to one's integrity enables one to live with oneself—to be at peace with oneself—to maintain one's self-respect.

Job was urged by his three counselors to join with them in their traditional views of God's rewarding the righteous and punishing the evil. He was inwardly pressured by his dread of the divine majesty to abandon his protest against God's injustice, for the proffered safety of conformity. It was *scary* to be out on his limb. Yet to retreat to the safety of the main trunk was also scary. He would lose his identity as he understood it. In his holding to his integrity under such duress, Job was living out his reputation for righteousness—"There is none like him on the earth." (1:8)

To facilitate or educe such integrity in counselees is a goal of counseling. Beyond the more immediate goals of al-

leviating current stresses and achieving interpersonal rec-
onciliations, the long-range goal is the spiritual growth of the
counselees—the development of the human under God. It is
ironic that Job's affirmation of his integrity should be the
outcome of the friends' counseling. Certainly this was not
their goal for Job's development. But in a perverse sort of
way their pressures on Job to conform were counterproductive with a person of Job's ego strength. They served instead primarily to stiffen his resistance. We need to ask,
however, what may have happened to one of lesser fortitude
under such counseling?

The third cycle of speeches, chapters 24–28, has a different structure than the previous two. The third speech of
Bildad is uncharacteristically short (6 verses) and there is no
third speech of Zophar to complete the poetic symmetry. In
addition, some of the material ascribed to Job sounds much
more like his counselors. Also in the midst of the speech
ascribed to Job are the words, "and Job again took up his
discourse" (27:1).

Although there are proposals for interpreting the
speeches as we have them, the conclusions of Old Testament
scholar Samuel Terrien seem to me to best account for these
difficulties. According to Terrien, chapters 24–28 have evidently undergone some damage or subsequent editing in their
structure in the manuscripts now available to us. He places
the section, 25:18–25 in a speech ascribed to Job (which the
RSV precedes with "You say" in order to refer them to the
three friends rather than to Job) as the beginning of the third
speech of Zophar. He ascribes 27:13–23, in a speech ascribed
to Job, as the conclusion of Zophar's speech. The remainder
of Bildad's speech would be 26:5–14. Job's speech about his
integrity (27:1–12) would then be in reaction to this second
part of Bildad's speech. Chapter 28 is an ode to wisdom which
most resembles the poetic style attributed to God in the theophany. Since this is a Christian caregiving study of *Job* and
not an exegetical commentary, it behoves us to move now
to Chapters 29–31, Job's final speech.

Chapter Seven

The Strength of Nietzschean Defiance

When Job takes up his discourse again he says nothing that is directed to the three counselors. Having affirmed his integrity in a defiant refusal to bow to their pressure to "toe the line," he now turns to reflecting on his life. His mind goes back to the "good old days" as a temporary respite from his present misery. He indicates his age by saying he was in his "autumn years." In the past he and God were *friends*. "The friendship of God was upon my tent" (29:4). In those days he took his place of respect as an elder in the gate. "When I went out to the gate of the city, when I prepared my seat in the square, the young men saw me and withdrew, and the aged rose and stood" (29:7–8). And why was he held in such esteem? "Because I delivered the poor who cried, and the fatherless who had none to help him" (29:12).

The "good old days" were probably never as good as they seem in retrospect. Memory has its own screening effect. Nevertheless, Job's description of his place in the community is consonant with the description of Job in the prologue. He continues in his memories. "Men listened to me, and waited, and kept silence for my counsel. ... I smiled on them when they had no confidence ... I chose their way, and sat as chief, and I dwelt like a king among his troops, like one who comforts mourners" (29:21,24,25).

1. Then and Now?

Chief! King among his troops! A far cry from his present status. *But now*! What an awful contrast! "But now they make sport of me." Who? Who would make sport of one who was once a chief and a king? "Men who are younger that I, whose fathers I would have disdained to set with the dogs of my flock" (30:1–2). Job's class-consciousness comes through. These were riff-raff—the dregs of society—"a senseless, a disreputable brood" (30:8). And these lowlifes dare to laugh in ridicule of the fallen chief. In derision they "spit at the sight of me" (30:10).

Job noted how people have no compassion for the mighty when they fall. Rather, they take the fall as an opportunity to release whatever resentment they have harbored (12:5). Now Job sees in their attacks a sadistic delight in the reversal of roles. These people on the socio-economic bottom of society, who were also younger than he, saw in Job an available target upon which to release their chronic anger. Job finds it humiliating being the brunt of their hostility. His sensitivities are outraged.

And who does Job hold responsible for all of this humiliation? God! God is the adversary who has "loosed my cord and humbled me." Because of this, "they have cast off restraint in my presence" (30:11). Job is their safe scapegoat. But it is *God* who "cast me into the mire" (30:19); it is God who "hast turned cruel to me; with the might of thy hand thou dost persecute me" (30:21). He wishes he could get some relief from his suffering—could retire to his bed, for example, and escape through sleep. But even then "the night racks my bones, and the pain that gnaws me takes no rest" (30:17). His miserable skin disease gives him no peace, night or day. For this too, Job holds God responsible.

Reflecting on the slow and cruel death of his wife, C. S. Lewis, like Job, laid the responsibility on God. "Month by month and week by week you (God) broke her body on the wheel whilst she still wore it." Job would have understood and would also have concurred with Lewis' conclusion. "The terrible thing is that a perfectly good God is in this matter hardly less formidable than a Cosmic Sadist" (*A Grief Observed,* Greenwich, Ct.: Seabury Press, 1963, p. 35). For the

Job of the poetic section, God has become like the Satan of the prologue.

Our images of God are influenced by our life experiences. The image that is formed in pain, and in the fear or terror connected with pain, may contain characteristics normally associated with the demonic—the cosmic sadist—the adversary. Lewis put it bluntly. "The tortures occur. If they are unnecessary, then there is no God or a bad one. If there is a good God, then these tortures are necessary. For no even moderately good being could possibly inflict or permit them if they weren't" (*A Grief Observed,* p.36).

Since it is torture, is it any wonder that Job cries out for help? "Yet does not one in a heap of ruins stretch out his hand, and in his disaster cry for help?" (30:24). Although the Hebrew in this verse is difficult, this translation fits the context. Necessary or not, Job believes his "torture" is undeserved. "Did not I weep for him whose day was hard? Was not my soul grieved for the poor? But when I looked for good, evil came; and when I waited for light, darkness came" (30:25–26). It was not at all what Job had expected for himself. On the basis of past experience he had assumed a different ending to his life. "I thought, I shall die in my nest, and I shall multiply my days as the sand ... my glory fresh with me, and my bow ever new in my hand (still vigorous in old age)" (29:19–20).

With that anticipation of providence, how depressing is the present misery. *But now* it all seems like a nightmare. Job's calamity is for him a sign of providence's betrayal. "My heart is in turmoil, and is never still; days of affliction come to meet me. I go about blackened, but not by the sun; I stand up in the assembly, and cry for help. I am a brother of jackals ... My lyre is turned to mourning, and my pipe to the voice of those who weep" (30:27–31).

Job is overwhelmed with self-pity. His account of what is going on within him is a description of the agitation of a person in depression. Although the depressed person looks phlegmatic and passive, his or her internal state is active in torment. This inner "turmoil" is so torturously active that it can lead one to look to suicide as a release—a way of stilling the torment. While Job has had a death wish, he has given no indication of being actively suicidal. Were he among us today in need of the help he kept asking for, we would probably observe that his ego strength was amazing for the amount of conscious pain he was enduring. We would be more moved by compassion to alleviate his pain than by fear that he would take his life.

2. Ministering to the Depressed

But others in a similar state of misery may be suicidal. In the spiritual care of a depressed person we need to keep alert to this possibility so that we can facilitate the precautions to prevent any self-destructive activity. The family of the depressed person needs to be aware of this possibility. Because of close connections to the families of troubled persons, the pastor and other Christian caregivers are in an excellent position to provide the guidance they need in taking precautionary measures. The working relationship with a local psychiatrist or psychiatric clinic comes in handy at these times. Besides the guidance that he or she can provide for the pastor in regard to the troubled person, the psychiatrist is the professional to whom the spiritual counselor can refer these persons for care. Consequently, it is wise for clergy and other Christian caregivers, as soon as they locate in a community, to ascertain the psychiatric as well as other therapeutic resources that are available and to begin cultivating a team relationship with these resources.

The most successful therapeutic approach for depressed persons is largely considered to be cognitive therapy. In contrast to a continuous reflection of feelings, the cognitive therapist attempts to challenge the thinking and belief systems of the depressed person. Obviously, if we interpret what happens in ways that are neither realistic nor healthy, we will generate by our interpretive system the feelings associated with depression. The idea behind cognitive therapy is to help the depressed person to establish beliefs that are rational as well as realistic, so that the thinking that stems from these beliefs will generate more positive feelings.

This actually is what the three counselors thought they were doing with Job. His interpretive system was bizarre to their way of thinking, so they tried to straighten him out in his believing and thinking. Job even concurred with some of their positions, and as we have noted previously, some of their teachings are found elsewhere in Scripture, though applied differently. But the three lost their bridge of empathy when they could not accept the exaggerated expression in Job's lament, and in its place they developed a defensive-offensive pose with Job that polarized their positions. Someone will have to re-establish an empathic relationship with Job, and through that relationship assist him to expand his cognitive awareness of the nature of life in a fallen world within the context of faith in God. This is the challenge before the fourth counselor.

But Job has not yet given full expression to what he believes and thinks. His "poor me" frame of mind has its counterpart in self-justification. Having concluded his lament over his miserable lot in comparison to the glory he once had, he now focuses on his blameless character.

3. Searching the Heart

Job had twice refuted Eliphaz' attack on his character by alluding to his acts of kindness, but now he is ready to give the attack his full attention. Perhaps it took a while for the initial hurt to subside and for his anger to come to the fore. Self-pity with its concomitant self-righteousness leads now to self-justification.

Job scrutinizes every aspect of his life and affirms his innocence in each. His is a full-scale rebuttal of every charge made against him—and more. The extremes in the attack bring on the extremes in the defense. Point by point, Job answers Eliphaz regarding his sexual life, both in fantasy and in reality, his treatment of his servants, his dealings with the poor, his attitude toward money, his attitude toward his ene-mies, and finally, his use of his land. In each instance Job declares himself innocent of the charges; to have been guilty would have meant being "false to God above" (31:28).

For Job, sexual morality begins within, in the mind and heart. "I have made a covenant with my eyes; how then could I look upon a virgin?" (31:1). Such inward lusting would have brought the displeasure of God, who not only sees his inner life but holds him accountable for it. "Does not he (God) see my ways, and number all my steps?" (31:4). What about his personal honesty? "If I have walked with falsehood, and my foot has hastened in deceit; Let me be weighed in a just bal-ance, and let God know my integrity!" (31:5–6). Nor has he coveted his neighbor's wife. "If my heart has been enticed to a woman, and I have lain in wait at my neighbor's door . . . that would be a fire which consumes . . . and it would burn to the root all my increase" (31: 9,12).

How did he treat those under him—his servants? "If I have rejected the cause of my manservant or maidservant, when they brought a complaint against me; what then shall I do when God rises up? . . . Did not he who made me in the womb make him? And did not one fashion us in the womb?" (31:13–15). One needs to be reminded of the time in which these words were written to realize how remarkable they are. Job recognizes that his servants have the right to complain against him, and he has the obligation to take their cause seriously. And why? Because both he and they are equal before God—equal at birth. Job's is a truly outstanding social consciousness, for his culture.

Since Job was sufficiently affluent to have servants, how did he treat the unaffluent—the poor? "If I have withheld anything that the poor desired, or have caused the eyes of the widow to fail, or have eaten my morsel alone, and the fatherless has not eaten of it . . . then let my shoulder blade fall from my shoulder . . . " (31: 16,17,22). And why was he so generous with his wealth? "For I was in terror of calamity from God and I could not have faced his majesty" (31:23).

Job describes himself as the best that the law of Moses can produce. His righteousness is a religious righteousness of law, and fear of the wrath of God is its motivation. And it was impeccable! Is it any wonder that Job who had behaved inwardly and outwardly so righteously to avoid calamity, would feel betrayed by God when he experienced calamity? But Job needs to have reinforced the religious righteousness of the Gospel with the love of God as its motivation.

Nor as an affluent man has he become a materialist by trusting in money. "If I have made gold my trust, or called fine gold my confidence; if I have rejoiced because my wealth was great, or because my hand had gotten much ... I should have been false to God above" (31:24,25,28). Job knew the potential idolatry in wealth and rejected it to be faithful to the true God.

As he harbored no secret satisfaction in his wealth, so he harbored no secret satisfaction in the misfortunes of his enemies. "If I have rejoiced at the ruin of him that hated me, or exulted when evil overtook him—I have not let my mouth sin by asking for his life with a curse" (31:29–30). By now Job has turned his search into every nook and cranny of his life. He has epitomized his culture's respect for hospitality. "The sojourner has not lodged in the street; I have opened my doors to the wayfarer" (31:32). So far as he is consciously aware, he has concealed nothing that is negative about himself. "If I have concealed my transgressions from men, by hiding my iniquity in my bosom, because I stood in great fear of the multitude, and the contempt of families terrified me, so that I kept silence, and did not go out of doors" (31:33–34). Nothing hidden, no facades, no hypocrisy, no fear of what people would think or say, no withdrawal from public exposure: Job's life is the proverbial "open book" for all to see.

4. Like A Prince
At this point Job breaks off his self-scrutiny. The RSV appropriately ends the final sentence with a —. It is as though Job realized the futility of his self-justification and were saying,

"Enough of this monologue about my innocence—I want a hearing!" "Oh, that I had one to hear me!" Here is my signature! Let the Almighty answer me!" (31:35). I'll sign this affirmation of innocence.

But say something, God! "Oh, that I had the indictment written by my adversary!" (31:35). Again God is presented as the adversary and accuser like the Satan of the prologue. And what would this self-proclaimed innocent man do with the indictment if he had it? "Surely I would carry it on my shoulder; I would bind it on me as a crown" (31:36). He is confident he can refute it. "I would give him an account of all my steps; like a prince I would approach him" (31:37). Like a prince! Job is anything but humbled; he holds his head high! Here is Nietzschean defiance: no groveling for grace. He'll take on the king like a prince—a peer!

At this point Job evidently recalls an area of his life that he forgot to examine. As a person of wealth, Job had much land. How had he used it? "If my land has cried out against me, and its furrows have wept together; if I have eaten its yield without payment, and caused the death of its owners; let thorns grow instead of wheat, and foul weeds instead of barley" (31:38–40). He has been a good steward of his land—a good ecologist. He has not acquired it by killing its rightful owners, and he has not failed to replenish it with nutrients after using it. With this final affirmation of innocence, Job concluded his speech: "The words of Job are ended" (31:40).

"So these three men ceased to answer Job, because he was righteous in his own eyes"(32:1). The three counselors had *had* it. If we were dramatizing the story, we would direct the three to use their hands at this point in making gestures of futility toward Job. Why should they bother talking any further? He was incorrigible! They were wasting their breath.

Job outlasted his counselors. Although there were three of them, he fought them all to silence. He is stronger at the end than at the beginning of their dialogues. But it is a strength of defiance. Their conversations had become heated arguments. Few of us quarrel gracefully, especially with our intimates. Job's defensiveness made him unattractive as a person and unbalanced in his perspective. This is what can happen to sufferers when they are not given the understanding and compassion they need. In his defiance, Job is vital and triumphant. Regardless of how wrong-headed he may be in some of his conclusions, he remains honest—honestly believing that what he says is right. He had retained his integrity.

But Job has also lost something. This is what defensiveness can do. Job is strong but inflexible, certain but isolated. He had won, but he had also lost. He still needs help. He has "hair on end" like a feisty cat. At this stage he is a far cry from the Job of the theophany. How does he get from here to there? Pastorally speaking, a transition is needed. Neitzschean defiance is something other than worship and adoration. It is not the "strength (that) is made perfect in weakness" (2 Cor. 12:9 KJV). The needed transition to God's speech comes in the ministry of Elihu.

Chapter Eight

The Value of Structuring

When "these three men ceased to answer Job, because he was righteous in his own eyes" (32:1), another counselor stepped into the fray. There has been no mention of Elihu until now, although he makes clear his prior presence by saying, "I gave you my attention" (32:12). Nor is there any mention of Elihu in the epilogue. He is a Melchizedek-like figure who enters unexpectedly and leaves without notice.

1. Whence Elihu?

From the perspective of pastoral theology and pastoral counseling from which we are exploring Job, Elihu is needed, as previously noted. The book hangs together in all of its parts. Some conjecture that this may be the result of an editor with both literary and human sensitivity skills. The writer of this section, as of the previous section, shows an intuitive awareness of dialogical dynamics. What we now perceive as modern insights into psychology, Christian care, and counseling have obviously tapped into an age-old wisdom regarding human nature and human behavior. I have been amazed to perceive this ancient wisdom, particularly in Elihu, that in our limited awareness, many believe originated in our time and place. I will focus largely on these strikingly modern processess and insights in this ancient piece of Wisdom literature.

2. An Angry Young Man

Elihu enters the conversation with an expression of respect. He had waited until now to speak because he thought those who were older would prove wiser. He was "young in years" (32:6), but he heard nothing that would move him to respect his elders. "It is not the old that are wise, nor the aged that understand" (32:9). He is an angry young man! But he is impartial in his disgust. He was angry at Job because he justified himself rather than God. And "he was angry also at Job's three friends because they found no answer, although they declared Job to be in the wrong" (32:3). Whatever had kept Elihu quiet according to the ageist tradition of his day was now overcome by his indignation at the folly of his elders as well as their ceasing to speak. "Therefore I say, 'listen to me; let me also declare my opinion' " (32:10).

3. Laying a Good Foundation

Elihu takes a rather lengthy route in sharing his opinions. For some commentators, he takes an overly-long time to get to the point. Actually, this time in getting to the point is a needed preparatory time. It is "setting the stage;" in modern counseling understanding, it is called "structuring the relationship." If we approach this story from a dramatic or even a human interaction point of view, Elihu is entering into the conversation when Job is already loaded with projections developed from what had gone on before. Why should he listen to Elihu if he was turned off by the others? Why would we anticipate anything different?

Based upon this interpersonal reality, Elihu moves quickly to dissociate himself from the three friends. "He (Job) has not directed his words against me, and I will not answer him with your speeches" (32:14). Perhaps Elihu sensed that if he was to penetrate Job's defenses, he needed to be a fresh voice. Otherwise, Job may have projected onto him the negative image he had developed toward the three friends.

Structuring the nature of a relationship when projections from the past could be a problem can make the difference between whether one is heard or not. The possibilities for a counseling relationship in these instances are largely determined by how one deals with these projections. Wives, for example, are more likely to come for pastoral marriage counseling than are husbands. The reasons for this lie in our culture's pressures on males to have it all together. But counselors know that to be effective in such instances, they need also to talk to the husband. In making the overture to such a reluctant husband, the pastor will need to do much structuring. After extending an invitation to George Stock to come with his wife Ellen for counseling, Pastor Johnson received the following reaction.

"I don't know what she is coming to you for. We can work out these problems by ourselves."

"I imagine it is somewhat embarassing to you that she has seen me," said the pastor, "but I'd like to assure you that she did so because she is really interested in your marriage, and my role is simply to help you both help yourselves."

George shot back quickly, "I don't think I need your help, pastor."

"That may be, George," said the pastor, "but I need yours. I really cannot be a competent counselor to Ellen when I only get her side of the story. I need yours to see it in balance."

"Yeah, I can imagine what she's told you."

"To be fair to Ellen," said the pastor, "I would have to say that she has shared a great deal of love for you. But I hear you. I've heard Ellen's side only, and so it might seem that I am already biased in the matter. Well, I'm not. I've been through enough of these experiences to know how subjective one can be when there's a problem. But beyond that, I am a *Christian* counselor—and this means I'm not an ally of Ellen in this marriage difficulty; rather, I am an ally only of the marriage itself.

"Okay," said George. "But what makes you think we need help?"

"For one thing, Ellen does. For another, I've needed help at times too. We can get so involved in these conflicts that it may take a skilled outsider to help us. It's no shame to admit needing help. In fact, it's to your credit. God didn't create us to be loners—but rather to be givers and receivers with others. That's why we have a church. I might be able to be of help, George."

"Let me think it over, Pastor. If I decide to come, I'll show up with Ellen next time."

"Why not talk it over with Ellen also," said the pastor, "I had her permission to invite you. In fact, she wants you to come. I'm no threat to you, George—actually, I'm your friend. And there are times when all of us need friends. And being a spiritual counselor is one way I can be a friend now to you both."

"Thanks, Pastor, for making the effort to contact me. I know I'm not easy to find. I promise you to consider it seriously."

George Stock was resistant to the pastor's invitation. His picture of what counseling would be like was far different from the pastor's. This discrepancy needed to be clarified. Also, as a male in our society, he was embarrassed at being exposed as needing help. His denial was his defense of his masculinity. This illusion of self-sufficiency needs also to be confronted in a gentle and yet persuasive way. Pastor Johnson may have had a lot of insights to offer George based on his session with Ellen, but he knew that George's openness to receive them depended on his wise structuring of their possible counseling relationship. The pastor's purpose in the structuring was to help George let down his defenses so he would allow himself to be open to what he needed and possibly even desired—to receive help for his marriage.

4. Identifying with the Other

Elihu believed strongly that he had something fresh to say. "Behold, my heart is like wine that has no vent, like new wineskins, it is ready to burst" (32:19). Therefore, "I must speak, that I may find relief" (32:20). He is honest enough to acknowledge his personal involvement. He is not detached. He is speaking for his own sake as well as Job's.

Yet Elihu evidently knows how important it is in entering this already heated arena to be impartial. "I will not show partiality to any person" (32:21). And why not? "Else would my Maker soon put an end to me" (32:22). This is the same motivation Job had given for his virtuous living (31:1–4). Elihu's appeal to a like motivation for his impartiality is now called *identifying* with the counselee.

A man whom I had come to know through professional gatherings asked me if I would contact his wife. Six months previously, they had experienced the sudden and tragic death of their teenage daughter. After the formal contacts that took place relating to the funeral, his wife had increasingly withdrawn from any social engagements. She spent her time sitting in her daughter's room, emerging only perfunctorily to prepare the evening meal and to retire to bed. But even then after tossing and turning she would frequently arise to return to the room. The husband warned me that she might refuse to see me.

When I called, the husband suggested I go directly to the daughter's bedroom since he had told her I would be calling. As I approached the room I called her name. She looked up with no semblance of a smile. "Your husband has told me of your tragedy and I have come as a pastor to offer my sympathy and to visit with you if you will permit me."

"I don't want to talk with anybody," she said.

"I can understand that," I replied.

"How would *you* understand!" she said with an impassive contempt.

"I just might," I said. "Someone very precious has been taken from you and you've lost interest in your life. This room is the closest you can come to her, and so you stay here." She neither looked up or said anything. "The future is bleak—if not impossible—to think about," I continued. "You would like to die right in this room." She looked at me intently but still did not speak.

"You are wondering how I know," I said. "Because I have been there. I too have lost a daughter to death. I know the despair, the death wish, not wanting to be with people—unable to tolerate their lighthearted talk."

This time she spoke. "And it gets worse instead of better."

"For a long time," I said. "May I come in?" She nodded. "You can sit on the bed."

Because I could identify with her, she began to see me as a companion rather than an intruder, and she let me in—to her life.

5. The Counselor's Congruence

Elihu's identification with Job's inner self not only helped Job to lower his defenses, but also provided an early basis for the establishment of rapport. After laying this good foundation Elihu asked Job to listen to him. "But now, hear my speech, O Job, and listen to all my words." And the reason? Elihu is congruent, authentic, genuine. "What my lips know they speak sincerely" (33:1–3).

In testing the effectiveness of his counseling methodology, client-centered therapist Carl Rogers discovered instead the effectiveness of the qualities of the counselor's person. The first of these is the counselor's *congruence.* If the counselor is a genuine person—sincere, with no hidden agenda of manipulation or control—the relationship is predisposed to be healing and constructive. Congruence means to be the same on one's inside as on the outside. The counselee need not wonder what the counselor is "up to." What Elihu had to say was coming from his heart. Job could trust his counselor.

A wise and veteran sufferer said, "Show an interest in me and my concerns, touch me, and I will listen to whatever you have to say." This is what Elihu was doing in his long introduction. He was "touching" a defiant, defensive Job so that he would let down his defense enough to listen to what Elihu had to offer him.

6. An Open Atmosphere

But Elihu still has more structuring to do. After his expression of genuine concern, he encouraged Job to continue to speak his mind. "Answer me, if you can; set your words in order before me; take your stand." (33:5). This atmosphere is to be open and dialogical. "Behold, I am toward God as you are; I too was formed from a piece of clay" (33:6). This is to be a dialogue between *peers*—equals as they stand before and under God. Therefore, "No fear of me need terrify you; my pressure will not be heavy on you" (33:7).

If we were dramatizing the Book of Job we could show Job's involvement at this point. The text gives us no indication except that Job is silent. Yet he is becoming open to receive where before he was not. The character playing Job could demonstrate Job's involvement non-verbally by responding with an amused smile to Elihu's "youngish" appeal to knowledge and sincerity. He could respond at the completion of Elihu's introductory structuring with a hand gesture that would indicate "go on."

By placing himself in the same place with Job and disavowing any tendency to coerce, Elihu is encouraging an accepting atmosphere, in contrast to that of the three friends. He will respect Job's space. These assurances of acceptance and openness must have sounded refreshing to Job's ears after his battle against the coercive guilt-tripping of the three friends.

Chapter Nine

Restatement: A Healing Process

After laying a good foundation in structuring this counseling relationship in impartiality and openness, Elihu is ready to make his first gesture, namely, to offer his understanding. He restates and reflects Job's position of feeling abused by God. "You say, 'I am clean, without transgression; I am pure, and there is no iniquity in me. Behold, he (God) finds occasions against me, he counts me as his enemy' " (33:9–10). Elihu is obviously showing this understanding from what he had heard. This is an accurate restatement of Job's expression of his position. In current counseling, the restatement or reflection is used to show the other that the counselor has heard—is following. It is a way of getting to know another person. It shows that the counselor is listening and therefore encourages continued communication from the counselee. Instead of saying, "I understand," a restatement of the counselee's expression in the counselor's own words *demonstrates* this understanding, and is much more convincing.

1. Reflecting in One's Own Words and Identification

A restatement is not a statement of agreement. It simply acknowledging where the other is in the context of his or her thinking, feeling, and desiring. Obviously Elihu does not agree with Job even though he can express the way Job feels. After his restatement he expresses his own point of view regarding it, which will be taken up in the next chapter.

Restatement or reflection is easy to comprehend as a method, and easy to caricature, but difficult to do in a personally involved way. Perhaps this is why it is so attractive to caricature. Carl Rogers' earlier non-directive or later client-centered counseling has taken the brunt of this caricaturing: "I'm feeling depressed." "Oh, you feel depressed." Or "I'm worried about my marriage," "I see, you are worried about it." These are examples of parroting rather than reflecting. A reflection is put into one's own words. Using the marvelous elasticity of language with our imaginative capacity, our conversational restatements can broaden the counselee's own understanding of what he or she has said.

While reflection appears as a simple method, it can be difficult to do if we allow ourselves to enter the world of the other. It temporarily puts the counseling process into a state of uncertainty which may be difficult for those who want to go right into a solution. The focus is on the problem rather than the solution. The counselor is challenged to live in the emotionally charged moment rather than to stay at a safe distance from it.

This raises the question of over-identification. One can so feel with the counselee that one takes on the problem as one's own. Obviously this is not going to be helpful since there will then be two who need help. As Rogers puts it, the counselor identifies with the inner world of the other *as if* it were one's own. The words *as if* are important because this inner world is not the counselor's. The counselee needs the support of the counselor who, while identifying with how the counselee feels, is also securely anchored in the world of objectivity. Of course, objectivity is difficult to come by, since we are all influenced by our own subjectivity in how we view reality. But since the counselor does not share the psychological state of the emotionally disturbed counselee, nor his or her interpretation of the context of the problem, the counselor is much more likely to have a better grasp on reality at that point. This the counselee needs from the counselor.

2. Coming to Peace with Shadows

This obligation requires a counselor who has come to peace in some measure with his or her own shadows or demons. We all have our darker side with its influence upon our inner and outer behavior. But through the assurance of the Gospel that God in Christ accepts us despite our darker side, we can come to peace with ourselves as we are. It is this peace that enables us to live constructively with our shadows, and to deal with the shadows of others.

With this basis for security, the counselor can take the risk of letting the air charge up and have the courage to accept the other's emotional state so that one can put its description into one's own words. In this way we face reality fully before trying to change it. As Soren Kierkegaard put it, if we are going to move from the spot where we are, we need to begin at that spot. The spot where we are is often so uncomfortable that we would rather deny it or distract ourselves from it.

It may be particularly hard to deal with the counselee's "spot" when it includes emotions of anger or despair, protests against God's ways, or even doubts about God's existence. There is a temptation to avoid dealing with these feelings, to defend God, or to try to talk the counselee out of the fact that they have these feelings and attitudes. But as previously mentioned, acceptance of such threatening communication, listening to what we naturally would rather not hear, builds the bridge of identification which God can use as a healing influence in the relationship.

Restatement is particularly effective with people who repress their hostility, despair, and other uncomfortable emotions and thoughts. Some have learned to preserve their relationship with others and even with God by denying they have these emotions. It is their habitual way of holding on, of surviving. They may seem easier to counsel than an angry Job, but actually they are more difficult to help. Everything may be sacrificed to preserve their precarious equilibrium, even their honesty and integrity. Kierkegaard was well aware of this safety procedure of not putting words to our disturbing thoughts and feelings. "One regrets ten times for having spoken, to once for having kept silent—and why? Because the external fact of having spoken can involve one in difficulties, since it is an actuality. But to have kept silent! And yet this is the most dangerous of all. For by maintaining silence, a person is thrown wholly upon himself. Here actuality does not come to his aid by punishing him, by heaping the consequences of his speaking upon him. No, in this respect it is easy to keep silent" (*Sickness Unto Death,* p. 34)

Job, on the other hand, valued his integrity more than his safety. The story of his integrity can be used to help people who are afraid to be honest. A hospital chaplain was concerned about one of his sufferers because she seemed discouraged but would not own up to it. When he gently inquired about her feelings, whether her illness was disturbing her spirit, she replied, "We are not supposed to feel that way." When the chaplain asked her where she had gotten this idea, she replied, "It is not Christian to feel that way—it doesn't show faith." The chaplain held her hand and said, "There is often a difference between what *should* be and what *is*—even in the hearts of Christians. God knows what *is,* and God in Christ loves us regardless. There is a person in the Bible that I am sure you have heard about—Job—who felt so secure with God that he told God in the strongest terms that he thought God was treating him unfairly in his sufferings. His friends thought that God would punish him, but instead God accepted his honesty. This honest relationship with God finally helped him to be at peace in his heart."

At this point she began to cry. "I do feel so abandoned—and wonder whether I have any faith." The chaplain responded, "It must be very hard lying here, day after day, wondering what is going to happen to you." While this is simply an excerpt from the visit for illustration, it is obvious that the chaplain now can pray with her in petitions that speak from her heart.

Job's opposite, the one who in Luther's words cannot "sin boldly," still has a "Job" within. This can be seen, for example, in the above patient. Although she expressed her protest in a more passive way, she is still protesting her lot. The counselor's challenge is to get the Job within to express him or herself. The Christian counselor is a symbol-bearer of the faith. As he or she establishes an accepting relationship, actively listens for clues to any potential negative within, and pointedly responds to what clues are perceived, the dynamics of the relationship extend to the divine/human system. This connection of the counselor with God in the mind of the counselee enhances the therapy of the process.

3. Limitations of Restatement

Reflection as a way of encouraging people to express their uncomfortable feelings has its limits with people whose anger is self-generated by the distorted way they interpret what is transpiring in their lives. These openly hostile people in psychological parlance have decidedly paranoid tendencies. To such persons a restatement of their anger may be interpreted as an agreement and reinforcement of their distorted position. They need an approach which, as non-threateningly as possible, raises questions regarding their interpretations. This actually amounts to sowing a doubt about their *rightness.* Job was so continuously overwhelmed by his sufferings and aggravated by his three friends that his mental state could at times be perceived as paranoid. This is why Elihu sensed he had first to structure the relationship in as non-threatening an atmosphere as possible before he could either restate Job's position or confront him concerning it.

4. Responding to the Difficult

What goes on within us as Christian counselors when we hear people say such things as, "I wonder why this is happening to me?" or "Why is God doing this to me?" or "It seems that I am being singled out as God's 'whipping boy'." Some of us have a natural tendency to *react* to such statements, that is, to emotionally pull back from them. We feel the inner pressure to explain or defend or in some way justify God's ways. On the other hand, if we have the courage to respond to such statements, that is, to move toward them, we can accept these persons where they are in their protesting, doubting, fearful selves. This courage can come from believing that our responding is in itself healing, even though such healing is not immediately perceived. On the other hand, our explaining, defending, and justifying of God may do more to quell our own anxieties than those of the counselee.

The following verbatim concerns a crisis which pastors and all spiritual counselors may encounter in their ministry to the sick. Richard Carter has just received the bad news that his cancer, which he had reason to hope would not return, had done so.

Carter: Thanks for coming over, pastor. I needed to talk to someone since, as I told you on the phone, I have had a return of my cancer.

Pastor: I'm sorry to hear that, Richard. I too had hoped your cancer had gone. I am not in your position, but I obviously can realize your great disappointment.

Carter: Right. And suddenly it is a different world.

Pastor: What has happened to your hope?

Carter: At first it really crashed, but it has come back a little. Maybe I can still make it.

Pastor: I gather from the way you said that, that it is not an unrealistic hope.

Carter: No, it isn't, but it is not bright either. It makes me want to cry.

Pastor: I suppose you have.

Carter: You bet.

Pastor: And why not?

Carter: Except that I end up feeling sorry for myself.

Pastor: Like you were getting the short end of the stick.

Carter: Right. I find it hard to pray then, pastor. Something blocks me.

Pastor: Maybe you are angry over this disappointment and subconsciously, at least, perhaps you are angry with God.

Carter: I don't feel angry, really—it is just that I don't want to talk to God.

Pastor: You don't want to get too close to God right now; you feel you're not ready for that.

Carter: No—we've nothing to say to each other right now.

Pastor: Perhaps you feel let down—like God has let you down.

Carter: It's hard to say that, Pastor, but yes, I guess I do.

This is not the end of the pastor's Christian care by any means, but it is a first step in being helpful. The pastor is helping Carter to face his disappointment and anger openly. While his own faith is shaken at the moment, Carter can know that the faith of others continues for him. While he finds it difficult now to pray, he can be assured the Spirit is praying for him "with sighs too deep for words" (Rom 8:26). The psalmist's self-searching question comes to mind: "Why are you cast down, O my soul, and why are you disquieted with me?" (Ps. 42:5). The pastor has helped Carter to do this questioning and searching as preparation for the psalmist's next step. "Hope in God; for I shall again praise him, my help and my God" (Ps. 42:11).

What this pastoral visit has accomplished is an honest communication of where the counselee is in his spirit and in his relationship with God. Should the pastor offer to pray with him in his present mindset—and I believe he should be offered this opportunity—the pastor can better intercede for Carter and pray empathetically with him. Normally, people like Carter want pastoral prayer and will say so. But if the offer is declined, the pastor needs to respect the decision without any further indication of judgment on it. We can always pray for others privately.

This is also a time for Christian counselors to share their faith, fully acknowledging that they are not in the same situation. In subsequent chapters we will see that this is precisely what Elihu did. Carter needs encouragement, as did Job, to continue to hope. At the same time he also will need the church's help in facing the reality that all of us face—though not so immediately and existentially, perhaps—namely, our own mortality. The Christian Gospel of resurrection and life with God through all eternity is the obvious resource for this help. But again, this help needs to be given in this dialogical setting of honest communication in which reflection plays an important role. The Christian counselor will want to know where the counselee *is* in regard to this hope so he or she can relate the message to the *real* person.

5. Drawing Out Rather Than Telling

A pastor brought a tape of his conversation with an elderly parishioner for me to critique. The pastor listened well until he asked the man if he thought much about death. The man laughed—nervously, I believe—and said, "Well, we all have to go sometime." The pastor responded by saying, "It's so good that we have our Christian hope in the resurrection to comfort us." The man replied, "yes." But what was he thinking? Did he really feel "good" about this hope? The pastor didn't give him the opportunity to say, since he was primarily concerned about saying what he thought pastors were supposed to say regarding death. Or perhaps it was his way of avoiding the possibility of hearing what he would rather not hear, so he told the parishioner what Christians are supposed to say, rather than drawing him out on what his thoughts and feelings actually were. Our doubts are a natural concomitant of faith, but we too often see them as a threat and take precautions to keep them from coming to the center of our consciousness. Careful listening and reflection can facilitate taking a direct look at what seems threatening. Then our faith has a chance to deal with it.

Chapter Ten

The Difficult Task
of Confrontation

Having restated Job's position, Elihu proceeded to disagree. "Behold, in this you are not right" (33:12). This assertion would currently be perceived as a *confrontation*. The word literally means to come together "forehead to forehead." Perhaps we would say, "eyeball to eyeball." In counseling it means saying something that the counselee may be avoiding and wanting not to hear. Yet the counselor believes it needs to be said if the counseling process is to move ahead. *Confront* is not the best word because it often implies defiance or even antagonism. Perhaps a more descriptive word would be *being direct*. David Augsburger suggests we change *confronting* to *"care-fronting."* Thus the counselor would be "forehead to forehead" with another because he or she cares about the other.

1. Elihu Answers Job

Elihu immediately softened his confrontation by adding, "I will answer you" (33:12). This is precisely what he said the three friends failed to do (32:12). Elihu is particularly concerned about Job's charge that God does not answer him. The problem may be in Job rather than in God. "For God speaks in one way, and in two, though man does not perceive it" (33:13–14). God may be speaking, but not in a way that Job would recognize and be prepared to hear. In dreams, visions of the night, and other ways, God may be communicating (33:15–16). But because Job is not open to hear in ways other than he has anticipated, he claims God is not speaking to him.

Elihu's "answer" to Job could be seen as his need to defend God. When a counselee is speaking negatively about God, there is always the temptation for the spiritual counselor to defend God. But usually the counselor then is responding to his or her own need rather than to that of the counselee. God needs no defending—by Elihu or any other spiritual counselor.

But Elihu's answer could also be an honest attempt to remove an obstacle in the way of Job's "hearing." And since Job's defensiveness has made him more rigid than flexible, Elihu's answer makes a lot of sense. What he is saying is that there may be another way of looking at Job's problem than the way in which Job is looking. If one can change one's *interpretation* of one's experience, one may change one's whole attitude toward it. What before was "invisible" now becomes visible.

This method of offering a different interpretation of the counselee's experience is called "reframing." The idea is that we can change the entire "picture" by putting a different frame on it. When this occurs, we respond differently in our feelings toward that picture. If God may be speaking in one way or in two, Job can still hope. By reframing this experience, Job may yet hear God speak.

2. Continuing the Dialogical Approach

The method of confrontation in counseling calls for the same sense of inner security in the counselor as the method of restatement. They are emotionally of the same genre, because both stem from the same empathic concern for the counselee. Responding by restating and reflecting communicates this empathy and builds rapport with the counselee. Confrontation may follow as in Elihu's counseling, but in the same spirit and attitude. There should be no "clash of gears" emotionally or intellectually in the counselor when going from reflecting to confronting.

Even as confrontation follows restatement, so restatement needs to follow confrontation. The counselor should be willing to listen after the confrontation. Elihu expressed this ability clearly when he said to Job, "Speak, for I desire to justify you" (33:32). In other words, "If my saying you are not right sounded like an attack, please be assured that it was not. I desire to justify you, not to put you down. I am on your side."

It is important to perpetuate the dialogical setting following a confrontation. The counselee needs to respond, even if defensively. His or her reaction should be expressed. This aids the counselor in avoiding the pitfall of a power struggle. The confronter appears to be on top, the confronted on the bottom. But this is only an appearance; the reality of the supportive relationship may need to be reaffirmed. Elihu described his peer-like relationship with Job when he said, "I too was formed from a piece of clay" (33:4). Allowing the counselee to come back into the conversation without judgment after the confrontation affirms this freedom from pressure.

A pastor shared with me how a confrontation handled without pressure became a point of enlightenment for him. His counselor asked him, "Bob, what do you do with your anger?" Bob looked surprised. "What do I do with it? I don't have any anger." The counselor simply responded with "Oh," and that was the end of it. Since Bob didn't have to defend his reactive denial, he couldn't get the question out of his mind. Soon it was *he* who was asking himself the question. This began his realization of the huge amount of anger he had been harboring under the disguise of more "acceptable" labels. Now he could *name* it. Now he could deal with it.

3. When and How to Confront

When should the counselor use confrontation? When it becomes clear that the counselee needs additional help in perceiving reality about him or herself and the situation. Obviously, it takes much listening and reflecting in the process to arrive at this decision. Elihu's confrontation came after he had listened to Job (32:12).

When a counselor decides to confront the counselee, how should he or she do it? Since the counselee needs confrontation, the counselor likely will meet resistance. Were there no resistance, the counselee would probably have received his or her enlightenment without confrontation. Consequently, the counselor needs to confront in a way that will minimize this resistance. Elihu prepared well for his confrontation of Job with understanding and rapport to influence a receptive attitude.

Beside this needed preparation, the manner of confrontation also is important in reducing resistance. The immediate purpose of the confrontation may be to present an insight that the counselee lacks, an alternative option which has not been considered, or a challenge to act when one has rationalized one's inaction, or to point out a wrongheadedness in interpretation as Elihu did, or to block an escape route that has frustrated the counseling process. But the ultimate purpose is always to stimulate and motivate the counselee to responsible behavior. With this in mind, the counselor must decide the form or degree to which he or she will confront. These degrees are illustrated in the following forms in which confrontation can take place.

a. A reflective question which the counselor "lets hang" rather than pursues. This was the form the counselor used with Pastor Bob. Denial comes easily with this approach—as Bob illustrated—but without a resulting power struggle. To a woman locked in an attitude of resentment toward a co-worker, for example, the counselor could ask, "Do you suppose that your co-worker is as threatened by you as you seem to be by her?" This form of confrontation is like sowing a seed and waiting for it to sprout.

b. Sharing an insight—"Here is how I see it." The counselor has the vantage point of seeing the problem more objectively than the subjectively involved counselee. Consequently he has the authority to say "what is coming through to me." To a frustrated mother, for example, he could say, "What I'm seeing is that you are more frightened than angry over the deterioration in your relationship with your daughter." The counselee can minimize the counselor's insight or take it seriously. In either case, the counselor lets the counselee decide. As with raising a question, sharing an insight is as often a way of sowing a seed as it is of opening the conversation to deeper levels.

c. Making a suggestion. A suggestion is more directive than sharing an insight. The counselor is in effect making a request. Such a suggestion can be given, for example, to break an impasse caused by a counselee's behavior. To a person who always leaves the room when any argument or friction is expressed, the counselor might say, "I'd like to suggest that the next time your wife begins to criticize you, see if you can stay in the room for at least five minutes. This will challenge your habit of withdrawal, allowing you to begin a constructive way of dealing with conflict." If the counselee shakes his head and says, "That would be very hard for me." the counselor does not equate hard with impossible. "I know—that's why I said only five minutes. I would like for you to give it a try and tell me about it at our next appointment."

d. A direct disagreement that elicits an immediate response. Elihu's confrontation of Job took this form: "In this you are not right." After counseling with a woman regarding the drinking problem of her husband, the pastor sensed that she did not understand "tough love" and was enabling her husband's drinking by continually covering for him. She acknowledged that she often called in sick for him at his job when he was drunk and gave the same excuse when people— even his family—called to visit. Yet she defended herself by saying, "What else can I do as his wife?" The pastor responded with this form of confrontation: "I don't agree that covering for him is your duty as a wife. Your husband needs help for his drinking problem and he may never get it if he is constantly protected from facing the consequences of his drinking." Although the wife was taken aback by this confrontation, she was better able to talk about what she really wanted for her husband.

While it may appear that confronting takes more courage than restating, the same kind of courage is needed for both.

Both restating and confronting may deal with negative feelings, the former drawing them out, and the latter eliciting them. In both reflection and confrontation, the counselor must be willing to respond to these feelings, as threatening as they may seem. In confrontation, the counselor initiates the expression of these feelings, rather than following their expression, but only because he or she has first been a good follower. In reflecting, the counselor in effect holds up the mirror to the counselee. In confronting, the counselor is attempting to remove obstacles from the counselee's vision so that he can see the mirror. Once the counselor has taken the initiative, he or she needs again to follow. As the proverb says, "The purpose in a man's mind is like deep water, but a man of understanding will draw it out" (Prov. 20:5). Both restating and confronting will assist a person of understanding to do this drawing out.

4. Counselor's Resistance to Using Confrontation

Confrontation is difficult for many pastors and other Christian counselors. Perhaps it is difficult for most other counselors as well. My students in pastoral counseling find confrontation the method they are most reluctant to use, even when appropriate, because of their emotional resistance. Confrontation "confronts" our need to please—our need for a comfortable and light ambience. We fear the disruption of a friendly atmosphere. It is the same fear that prevents people generally from being honest. Why risk eliciting negative emotions from others when keeping quiet allows one to keep the ties comfortable? Congenial pastors, for example, may become so bound to their congeniality that they are hindered from being facilitators for growth. Some of us are better at passive listening in counseling than at active involvement. But passive listening is not listening in the care-giving sense of the term. For this reason the term *active* listening is often used to describe listening manifested by verbal responses to feelings. Passive listening may elicit conversation from those who talk easily, but it may not result in therapeutic encounters.

We need the willingness to risk the creation of "waves" for the caring and loving that motivates confrontation. I assigned to one of my students a request from a pastor that we call on a parishioner of his who was in a mental hospital. The student and the parishioner were the same age and met together weekly during the quarter. The student knew from his supervisor at the hospital that the patient was avoiding any conversation about his family relationships. When the student would broach the subject, the patient immediately found some reason to break off the visit—the need for the bathroom, a smoke, or that he had another engagement. The student was frustrated with this compulsive escapism and, after consultation with me, decided that he would confront the patient. When the patient again voiced his need to leave, the student said, "John, I don't want you to leave. I want you to stay and talk about this painful subject. I want to see you get well so you can leave the hospital—that's why I want you to deal with your pain." The patient must have heard the passion in his voice. He said, "You care, don't you!" "Of course I care," said the student. "Why do you think I keep coming to see you?" "I thought you were just doing your assignment," the patient replied.

The student's confrontation communicated his caring when nothing else had. It "opened the door." The student's sharing of his concern is not dissimilar to Elihu's confession to Job. "I must speak, that I may find relief" (32:20). Both show the counselor's personal investment in the relationship.

5. The Value of Seeing the Relationship

Seeing the counselee in action with others often gives the counselor another view of the problem. This happened when Pastor Rohde finally succeeded in getting Bill Carlson to bring his wife along for marriage counseling. Previously in his conversation with Bill, the pastor had the impression of a husband frustrated with a non-responsive wife. When Mary Carlson came she was non-responsive, but largely because Bill did most of the talking. When she did not accompany him on the next visit, the pastor decided to explore with Bill what he had observed.

Bill: "She wouldn't come this time. She just said she didn't want to. But at least now you have seen how she is."

Pastor: "What do you mean?"

Bill: "Well, you know. She just sat here—didn't contribute much—like always."

Pastor: "Yes, I did notice that. But I also noticed something else I'd like to share with you."

Bill: "What's that?"

Pastor: "You did most of the talking."

Bill: (pause) "I know. But what else can I do when she doesn't say anything?"

Pastor: "I know, Bill. And I attempted to engage her in conversation. But you came in before she did."

Bill: "Well, somebody has to say something.".

Pastor: "Bill, believe me, I'm not trying to be critical. But there were a couple of times when I'll admit that I was annoyed. I would ask Mary a question—and you would answer it."

Bill: "Did I? I wasn't aware of that."

Pastor: "I didn't think you were, Bill—and that's why I'm bringing it up. Maybe you need to hold back and give her more space."

Bill: (pause) "I don't know what to think. What you're saying hurts—but—(pause) I've occasionally wondered whether I'm not too much for her—but I don't like to think that."

Pastor: "Have you any idea why that thought bothers you?"

Bill: (pause) "Yeah—I'm afraid I do. (pause) I'm too much like my Dad, I guess—with my Mom. He just takes over. I used to get so mad at her—especially when I was still living at home—for not standing up to him."

Pastor: "You think maybe you picked up some of those traits?"

Bill: "I would never want to admit to that—it's scary. He's all that I *don't* want to be."

Obviously Pastor Rohde's confrontation created a tense moment in the counseling, but because of the backlog of rapport and his willingness to listen and be supportive to Bill, Rohde unearthed a significant "shadow" in Bill that could now be brought into the light.

6. God's Purpose Is Always Redemptive

Elihu's immediate offer to give Job an explanation and an alternative helped to soften the bluntness of his confrontation. "Your neck is stuck, Job, and if you loosen it so that you can look in all directions, you will have a wider perspective—you will see and hear things differently. Something may be going on in that silence. God may be speaking even though you are not aware of it."

And why may God speak in these other ways, "though man does not perceive it?" "That he (God) may turn man aside from his deed, and cut off pride from man; he keeps back his soul from the Pit, his life from perishing by the sword" (33:17–18). Here throughout his speeches, Elihu sees God's actions as redemptive and not punitive. God is doing it *for* Job. Like Elihu, God is on Job's side.

7. Acting from Wisdom rather than Annoyance

Too often confrontation comes from frustration and annoyance. Even if our words themselves don't show it, the counselee picks up the attitudes behind them. The confrontation then comes off as an attack. Confrontation may be associated with attack because it too often comes after the counselor has not faced his or her feelings of frustration and annoyance with the counselee. The signs of this are present when the counselor feels resistance as the time for the counselee arrives. He feels stuck in the relationship—the counseling process has reached an impasse—and he really doesn't want to have another session. In this attitude toward the counseling, the counselor's tolerance of his own restraint can be pushed too far, and the annoyance may come out impulsively as a confrontation. It is what the counselor had wanted to say previously, but lacked the will, the permission, to say it. Now the increased annoyance gives the permission, and the confrontation is colored by anger. In that sense it *is* an attack.

How much better to confront when the motivation is care and the guidance is wisdom. The words then carry the care, and the counselee responds differently than when the confrontation is an attack. Our spiritual wisdom and personal caring are sufficient permission to confront. Then the context is the most favorable for the method's effectiveness. We can speak the truth in love and be aware of the presence of God as we do it.

Chapter Eleven

Sharing an Insight

When Elihu said that God speaks in various ways to us in our sufferings for the specific purpose of delivering and redeeming, he had a definite picture in mind of how this redemption works in human experience. It was this insight that he wanted to share with Job. "Man," he says, "is also chastened with pain upon his bed, and with continual strife in his bones" (33:19). The description of suffering that follows fits Job, although it is *generic* man that is the subject. "His flesh is so wasted away that it cannot be seen; and his bones which were not seen stick out" (33:21). In identifying suffering with humanity and not with particularly sinful individuals, Elihu removed from Job the stigma that the three friends had placed on him.

1. The Envisioning of Deliverance

In contrast to these friends, Elihu identified himself (a man) with Job's predicament. He identified himself also with Job's hope. "If there be for him (the suffering individual) an angel, a mediator . . ." (33:23). In contrast to the three friends who never responded to Job's longing for a mediator, Elihu identified with it. This mediator would be *gracious* to the sufferers and deliver them from going down to the Pit by providing a *ransom* (33:24).

Elihu envisions the deliverance. "Let his flesh become fresh with youth" (33:25). Besides the bodily regeneration, there is also restoration to communion with God. "Then man prays to God, and he accepts him, he comes into his presence with joy" (33:26). The sufferer testifies to his deliverance. "He sings before men, and says, 'I sinned, and perverted what was right, and it was not requited to me' " (33:27).

The sufferer's restoration leads to his confession. God's

forgiveness precedes the sinner's repentance. Repentance, in contrast to despair, is sorrow with *hope*. The hope is for forgiveness. "He (God) has redeemed my soul from going down into the Pit, and my life shall see the light" (33:28).

Elihu's vision of the sufferer's deliverance is not something that happens only once in one's life, but is a repeated experience. "Behold, God does all these things, twice, three times, with a man, to bring back his soul from the Pit, that he may see the light of life" (33:29–30). This is Elihu's hope for suffering humanity, and, consequently, Elihu's hope for Job. This description of God's way of redemption is reflected in the New Testament picture of sanctification, patterned after the redemptive activity of Christ—the New Testament *ransom* for the sins of all (Mark 10:46; 1 Tim. 2:6). Spiritual growth after Baptism is a continuum of dips and rises, with the dip described as the crucifixion of the old nature and the rise described as the resurrection of the new nature (Romans 6:6–8). We shall pursue this correspondence between the Old and New Covenants regarding the Book of Job in the next chapter.

2. The Expertise of the Spiritual Counselor

Elihu's sharing of an insight is the second (b) of the milder forms of confrontation described in the previous chapter. His insight into God's redeeming ways offered a reframing for Job's experience of suffering. This is what Elihu believed he had to offer Job—and he wanted very much to share it.

Eliphaz had come close to this insight into God's role in human suffering in his first speech, particularly when he perceived Job's sufferings as a chastening experience. "Behold, happy is the man whom God reproves; therefore despise not the chastening of the Almighty. For he wounds, but he binds up; he smites, but his hands heal. He will deliver you from six troubles; in seven there shall no evil touch you" (5:17–19).

Like Elihu, Eliphaz had seen a positive outcome for suffering, but in contrast to Elihu, Eliphaz said the sufferer was still guilty, and God reproved and smote. Job, however, was not ready at that point even for a chastening understanding of his suffering, and he resisted it. Eliphaz and the others then went on the offensive to the extent that in his third speech, Eliphaz accused Job directly of gross sin (33:5–7).

Elihu's sharing is a model of what spiritual counselors have to offer those whom they counsel. The spiritual counselor's emphasis, as well as expertise, is in the spiritual dimensions of human problems. This expertise is offered in three specific areas.

a. *Sharing a Gospel Approach.* The spiritual counselor is equipped to give a Gospel approach to the counselee's need. Like Elihu, the counselor functions within the perspective that suffering is not necessarily sent by God as punishment for sin, even for such verbal expressions of defiance as Job's. Suffering is part of human experience in a fallen world, and God's role in this suffering is to use it redemptively for the sufferer. God is at work in our sufferings for our deliverance, our redemption, and our growth in perceiving the genuine values of life.

Like Job, sufferers still tend to search their lives, wondering if something they have done is the cause of their suffering— something over which they should feel guilt. Of course, some things we do or have done can cause subsequent suffering. There is a correspondence between lifestyle and health in body, mind, and spirit, and in our relationships. But God's ultimate goal in the suffering is not to "rub this in," even when such may be the case. Rather, it is to use the suffering for deepening the sufferers' capacity to develop the great potential for living with which God has endowed them.

Should the sufferer raise this question with his or her caregiver—whether God may be punishing—the caregiver needs first to draw the person out. "What specifically comes to your mind that might be something you are being punished for?" Confession is always good for the soul—and for healing. Let the guilt be expressed. Then the caregiver can communicate the Good News of forgiveness by grace for what has been confessed. The caregiver can move now to God's goal in the suffering. "God wants to assure you that you have his full forgiveness for all of these things. As you can see in Jesus Christ, God's love is absolutely unconditional. God is not judging you in your sufferings. Rather, God is here to help you—to be your friend—your healer." Words such as these, coming from the authority of a counselor of the church, challenge the law-oriented picture of God that sufferers bring with them or easily develop. The law picture is replaced by a Gospel picture—a genuine reframing.

b. *Knowledge of the Human Sciences.* Pastoral as well as other spiritual counselors are also educated in the human sciences of psychology and social psychology. They are alert to the interactions of feelings, intellect, and will, and also of what goes on between individuals in their significant relationships— the family and other systems within which we live that influence our functioning. While sharing insights in these areas may not be specifically religious in vocabulary, they are broadly religious in that they deal with God's creation of humanity.

One of the problems spiritual counselors have with marriage and family conflicts is that too frequently only one person comes for counseling. But counselors can compensate to some extent for this deficiency by their understanding of how our relational systems operate. Linda, for example, in her marital conflict, spent most of her time in the counseling telling how inconsiderate her husband was. The counselor knew that after the initial and necessary expression of this resentment, its continuous repetition could delay progress in achieving what Linda really wanted. So the counselor shared his concern with Linda. "We don't have your husband here, and so I don't know how he feels about these things. But I do know that you and your husband influence each other by how you relate to each other. So since we have you here, let's look into how you 'come off' to him. All of us can improve, and if you can make some changes in how you relate to him, we may influence how he relates to you."

c. *Pastoral Wisdom.* What accumulates from the counselor's experience is called pastoral wisdom—whether clergy or lay. The counselor's own faith journey in relating to God, self, and others also contributes to this wisdom. As we learn from experience, we can pass this pastoral wisdom on. Dave, for example, had a difficult time with his emotions, suffering from anxiety attacks that left him dysfunctional. Dave believed in God but said he was not able to pray for help. "I can pray for my family and friends," he said, "It's just that I don't feel right in praying for myself." "Would you like to receive God's help in your anxieties?" the counselor asked. "Sure, but how do I get it?" said Dave. "Ask for it. Jesus said 'Ask that you may receive.' God wants you to pray for yourself, in your need. There need be nothing difficult about this—it is simply admitting your need for God's help." "But how do I do it?" David demurred. "How would you ask me for help?" the counselor asked. "I don't know—just ask!" said Dave. "Right on!" said the counselor. "So think of God as a good friend, Dave. If you want God's help, then say so—God help me." With Dave's consent, the counselor closed the session with prayer in which he modeled for Dave in his intercessory prayers of petition. Then he encouraged Dave to close the prayer by honestly asking for what he wanted.

3. The Art of Maintaining a Dialogue

Having shared his insight on God's redemptive activity, Elihu asks for Job's response. "If you have anything to say, answer me" (33:32). To encourage Job, Elihu assures him that he is not an adversary (33:32). It is important for counselors to elicit a response once they have shared an insight. Otherwise, the dialogue may become a monologue, with the counselor resorting to repeating to reinforce the insight. These repetitions weaken the sharing, rather than strengthening it.

There is an art to retaining a dialogical setting following the sharing of an insight. The tendency is to stay in the role of the giver—the explainer. Our resistance to returning again to a dialogical pattern is again a matter of control. If the counselee seems to be accepting the insight, the counselor may feel secure enough to relinquish control. Otherwise, we may be moved to repeat ourselves to get the assurance we need.

It is one thing to *want* this assurance; it is another thing to *need* it. Since sharing an insight is a form of confrontation, as with other forms of confrontation, it is difficult for the counselor to stop the confrontation until he or she gets a consensus, and even this may only encourage more of the same because of the momentum of staying in control. The counselor is doing the talking, while the counselee is doing the head-nodding. This tendency to continue too long in the sharing role can be controlled when the counselor realizes that he or she is being propelled by the *counselor's* need, rather than the *counselee's.* So it is important for counselors to return to a dialogical milieu once they have shared the insight. "How does this seem to you?" the counselor may ask. There is a risk in doing this, of course, because the counselee's response is uncertain. So, therefore, is our control. What we need is trust in the God who is still with us in the uncertain, to take this step back into dialogue.

Genuine consensus will come more surely with the freedom of dialogue than with the coercion of monologue. Also, in asking for a response, the counselor has the opportunity—otherwise missed—of clarifying misunderstandings should they be expressed. Words can be precarious in that counselor and counselee may have two different interpretations of the same key word in the sharing of the insight. It is only as we encourage feedback that we may realize that we are not always as clear to others in our communication as we think.

So different from that of the three friends, Elihu's approach must have been refreshing to Job. So vocal before, Job now evidently preferred to listen instead. He'd had his say.

4. Songs in the Night
In what follows (chap. 34), Elihu seems to get carried away by his success in communicating. He takes to God's

defense with an intensity reminiscent of Eliphaz. But he returns again to deal honestly with Job's complaints. He had more to offer—another insight into Job's suffering.

As before, he began by restating Job's position. "You ask, 'What advantage have I? How am I better off than if I had sinned?' " (35:3). This restatement hearkens back to Satan's question in the prologue: "Does Job fear God for naught?" (1:9). It is at the heart of Job's lament. The three friends had avoided the question because it threatened their cause-and-effect understanding of the universe, as if God always in this life punished sin and rewarded obedience. So Elihu not only says he will give Job an answer, but also "your friends with you" (35:3–4). Perhaps Elihu had the courage to restate Job's threatening question because it was not as threatening to him as to the three friends. At any rate, in contrast to the three, he accepted the question as valid.

Elihu began his answer by noting Job's tendency to anthropomorphize when referring to God. Elihu says in effect, "Your wickedness and your righteousness (the subject of the long arguments between Job and the three) concern people like yourself. If you have sinned, what do you accomplish against him (God)? . . . If you are righteous, what do you give to him?" (35:6–7). In other words, you are focusing on the wrong level. In theological terms, Job and the three had been locked into the categories of the law, and the answer to Job's question is in the Gospel.

Elihu had something to say to Job's lamenting question. Job *was* "better off" for his covenanted life. Beginning with Job in his pain, Elihu said, "Because of the multitude of oppressions people cry out; they call for help because of the arm of the mighty" (35:9). When the arm of the mighty is the arm of the Almighty, this is a description of foxhole religion. The observation was made in World War II that there were no atheists in the foxholes (the holes where soldiers hid from enemy shelling). When people are distressed, they call for help to the One who is bigger than they.

Elihu contrasts this knee-jerk religiosity to the spirituality of those covenanted to God. "None says, 'Where is God my Maker, who gives songs in the night?' " (35:10). By putting the contrast into extremes—'People cry out' vs. 'None says'—Elihu uses hyperbole to make his distinction. In contrasting a spiritual person with an unspiritual person, Elihu anticipates St. Paul's similar differentiation. "The unspiritual man does not receive the gifts of the Spirit of God, for they are folly to him, and he is not able to understand them because they are spiritually discerned." (1 Cor. 2:14).

"Songs in the night," is a biblical metaphor for joy in the midst of trouble. The night hours are times of fear. Depressed persons fear the 4:00 a.m. hour when they awake to their terrors. The subconscious breaks through then into the conscious. The night—and the act of going to sleep—are also symbols of death and dying. Those who have songs in the night are no longer traumatized by the night.

The spiritual person is not one who simply cries out for help when in trouble. Rather, he or she believes also that God can sustain and strengthen in the midst of the trouble. It is this expanded insight into God's ways that Elihu sees as the advantage of the believer in times of trouble. The advantage is this capacity of the believer for a different kind of prayer when distressed than the simple cry for help—the capacity for prayer that values and asks for "songs in the night." Elihu's description of this advantage of the believer—the covenanted person, the spiritual person—is a prolepsis of what Job will himself experience in the coming theophany. The night will remain dark, but there will be peace and joy in the midst of it.

5. A Deeper Understanding of the Divine-Human Relationship

In his metaphor of "songs in the night," Elihu presents a deeper understanding of prayer than simply as a way of getting God to give us what we want. This in no way demeans prayers of petition—asking God for what we want. This we not only are moved to do in our distresses, but also are encouraged to do in the Scriptures. But along with this prayer for relief in our distress, there is in the spiritual person's petitions the awareness also that God will be with us even if the distress is not lifted—that God will "see us through" regardless of what happens.

The Old Testament scholar Samuel Terrien calls this insight of Elihu into songs in the night "one of the loftiest passages of the book, and indeed of the whole Bible" (*Interpreters Bible,* Nashville: Abingdon, 1980, vol. 3, p. 1152). Elihu sees this wider picture of God's influence in the time of trouble as a source of peace and joy. His focus is on the state of the soul.

Psychologist and philosopher William James' concept of the "inner door of consciousness" is helpful in understanding "songs in the night." It is at this inner door—where our spirit opens to the transcendent, interfaces with the Spirit of God— that, in the words of St. Paul, "the Spirit himself (is) bearing witness with our spirit that we are children of God" (Rom. 8:16).

With this larger understanding of God's help, the night becomes less threatening. God is there also. Folliott Pierpoint's marvelous hymn captures this perspective.

> For the wonder of each hour of the day and of the night;
> Hill and valley and tree and flow'r, sun and moon and stars of light:
> Christ our Lord to you we raise, this our sacrifice of praise.

This is the gratitude that comes from knowing that we are in God's hands—in the hours of the night—and that those hands are *good.*

Recently I encountered a former student who is now a parish pastor. When I asked him how things were going, he told me of the difficult conflict he had been enduring in his congregation. He had found himself the scapegoat for some of the disgruntlement certain persons had with the church. "We had a council meeting when all these things came to a head," he said. "I didn't sleep for nights before that meeting and for nights afterward." "I'm sorry to hear that," I said. "It must have been very hard on you." "It was—and it is," he replied, "but I'll tell you one thing—it sure draws you closer to God. You learn to trust that God is in the midst of it all—and it helps." "You're sleeping now?" I asked. "Yes," he said. He obviously had learned about "songs in the night."

Nothing could illustrate Elihu's insight into Job's agonizing question more than what actually happened to Job when the Lord answered him "out of the whirlwind."

Chapter Twelve

A Change from Within

After giving his answer to Job's question, Elihu turns his attention from Job to God. He invites Job to join in this change of focus and to reflect with him on the marvels of God's creative ways. It is as though he were taking Job's hand so that the two of them together could look to their Creator for the ultimate answer to Job's—to man's—predicament. And it is in nature as God's handiwork that Elihu sees the clue to this understanding. It is the arena in which the creature visibly perceives the Creator.

1. The Voice out of the Whirlwind

"Can any one understand the spreading of the clouds, the thunderings of his pavilion?" (36:29). Why does God do all of these marvelous and often fearful things? Again, Elihu sees God's ways, even in nature, as positive and redemptive. "Whether for correction, or for his land, or for love, he causes it to happen" (37:13). That God's purpose in all that God does is love points forward to the denouement in the coming theophany. Yet before, there is correction. Is Job so sure he wants his day in God's court? "Shall it be told him (God) that I would speak?" (37:20). Again, Elihu anticipates Job's reaction to the theophany. Elihu's theological perspective predisposed him to a different approach than the three friends; his hope for a mediator protected him from assuming he knew all there was to know.

"Then the Lord answered Job out of the whirlwind" (38:1). Finally Job hears God speaking. But what happened to Elihu? There is no closure such as "the words of Elihu are ended." Is Elihu still speaking? God's approach in the whirlwind is but a continuation of where Elihu was leading. Yet Job is now hearing God.

This lack of any line of demarcation between Elihu's ministry to Job and Job's encounter with God is a model of effective Christian counseling. The pastor and other spiritual counselors are the midwives to their counselees' own involvement—priesthood—with God, and when this involvement takes place, the counselor fades from the scene. When John the Baptist pointed his followers to the Lord, he modeled this same pastoral way. "He must increase, but I must decrease" (John 3:30).

Job had envisioned his encounter with God as one in which he would question God. Yet in the whirlwind (symbolic of Job's inner storm?), it is God who questions Job. "Gird up your loins like a man, I will question you, and you shall declare to me" (38:3). Job's encounter had come, but it is God who sets the agenda. God will question Job regarding the wonders of his creation.

"Where were you when I laid the foundation of the earth?" (38:4). "Or who shut in the sea with doors, when it burst forth from the womb?" (38:8). "Have you entered the storehouses of the snow?" (38:22). Now we look at these storehouses of the snow and see under the microscope the myriad of designs, intricate and symmetrical. "Who has begotten the drops of dew?" (38:28). "Can you bind the chains of the Pleiades?" (38:31). "Can you send forth lightnings?" (38:35). "Can you hunt the prey for the lion?" (38:39). "Do you know when the mountain goats bring forth?" (39:1). "Who has let the wild ass go free?" (39:5). "Do you give the horse his might?" (39:19). "Is it by your wisdom that the hawk soars?" (39:26).

The ostrich is a different object of marvel. She can outrun a horse (39:18), and yet is so stupid that she leaves her eggs on the ground where they can be trampled (39:15). She seems to have the wrong motherly instincts in protecting her young (39:16). Does God also have problems with creation?

2. Overwhelmed and Silenced

By this time Job's mind must have been reeling. Now God gives him the opportunity he said he wanted—his chance to question God. "He who argues with God, let him answer it" (40:2). But the defiant Job is no longer defiant. "Then Job answered the Lord: 'Behold, I am of small account; what shall I answer thee? I lay my hand on my mouth. I have spoken once, and I will not answer; twice, but I will proceed no further'" (40:3–5). Having put his "foot in his mouth," he will say no more. He is overwhelmed by this contemplation of creation and heavy questioning, and is silenced.

Evidently Job's silencing was not God's ultimate purpose. So the questioning began again, and as before, about the wonders of creation. "Have you an arm like God, and can you thunder with a voice like his?" (40:9). "Behold, Behemoth, [the hippopotamus] which I made as I made you; he eats grass like an ox. Behold, his strength in his loins, and his power in the muscles of his belly" (40:15–16). The other creature singled out is Leviathan (the crocodile). The description of Leviathan has a playful ambiance. "Can you draw out Leviathan with a fishhook, or press down his tongue with a cord? Can you put a rope in his nose, or pierce his jaw with a hook? Will he make many supplications to you? Will he speak to you soft words? Will he make a covenant with you to take him for your servant for ever? Will you play with him as with a bird, or will you put him on leash for your maidens?" (41:1–5). This lighter touch of humor could indicate the change that Job would experience in his perspective of God in this second part of the theophany.

The focus on these two creatures in this second revelation from God is probably because both of them have spiritual significance. The descriptions go beyond the normal hippopotamus and crocodile. Behemoth "is the first of the works of God" and cannot be captured (40:19, 24). Leviathan also cannot be captured (41:1), and appears like a dragon with fire coming from its mouth and smoke from its nose (41:19–21; cf. also Is. 27:1).

3. A Different Response

As the description of Leviathan concludes, Job breaks his silence. "Then Job answered the Lord: 'I know that thou canst do all things, and that no purpose of thine can be thwarted' " (42:1–2). Job had perceived the Creator in the creation. This enabled him also to see himself. " 'Who is this that hides counsel without knowledge?' Therefore I have uttered what I did not understand" (42:3).

Job's integrity is still intact. He had spoken what he believed was true. But he no longer sees things in the same way. His experience in the whirlwind changed his way of interpreting what had happened to him. He regrets what he said, and his question is reframed.

Job is changed from within. He saw things differently—his mind was changed. This is why he repented, for repentance is literally a change of mind. His perspective—his way of interpreting, of seeing himself and his surroundings—had changed because for Job, God had changed. Obviously, God had not changed, but Job's *picture* of God had changed. This change then changed the system between God and Job, which means Job too would change. This change is shown in his changed response. Since Job was seeing God differently, he saw himself differently. His relational system with himself had changed, and he repented.

Recently a friend of mine endured a debilitating illness. When I saw him, he said he was grateful for the illness. When I asked why, he said that he could see things now that before he couldn't see. When I asked for an example, he said, "I've always assumed my wife loved me, but now I know. I've seen her care in response to my illness, and now I have a deeper appreciation of her than I have ever known."

A change from within comes when the vehicle for change is love. Then it is an expression of freedom. This is why the Gospel changes us. When we receive God's revelation of forgiving and unconditional love, it changes us from the inside. In contrast, a change brought about by pressures from without, as represented by Law, curbs our freedom. Because it comes from without—through threats and coercion—it creates its own resistance, which is the only expression of freedom left. Job describes his change in perspective—a Gospel change from within—in words specifically describing his new relationship with God.

4. Mine Eyes Have Seen Thee

Having expressed his new understanding of God and of himself, Job's quest for answers may go on, but no longer out of the agony of alienation. The questions are reframed. From where does this renewed confidence and peace come to one who had been in such turmoil? Obviously, from his new awareness of who God is. "I had heard of thee by the hearing of the ear, but now my eye sees thee" (40:5). Job compares the first-hand knowledge of seeing with a second-hand knowledge of hearing. What had Job seen that so changed him? Not a God of power and majesty who silenced him! Rather, Job sees the God who loves him—who forgives him—who accepts him as he is—who is gracious to him and delivers him from the Pit. So he is not only freed from his fear of God's anger—he is free also to look candidly at himself. Since the fear of judgment is gone, he is able to repent. "Therefore I despise myself and repent in dust and ashes" (42:6).

A change in one system—Job with God—leads to a change in a closely related system—Job with Job. Who is the self he despises? Of what is Job repenting? As he looks back on his defiance of God, he sees how one-sided was his vision. He was seeing only in one way, rather than in two (37:14). He probably even feels foolish now about what he had said. But it does not matter. Job is at peace with God, and with himself. His repentance is evidence of his security with God. Only the secure repent and believe; the insecure defend themselves.

Is this the same Job whose pains were driving him to despair and defiance? What accounts for the difference? Job now has "songs in the night" (35:10).

The night continues, but he has received the resources to endure. In the midst of his troubles, rather than in their removal, Job had triumphed over his despair. He still does not know why he is suffering, but the question no longer torments him. He now *sees* what before he had only heard about. What he saw—the God of love—now enables him to trust, though he still does not understand.

Psychiatrist Viktor Frankl maintains that we humans have a basic need for meaning and purpose for our survival. He quotes Nietzsche, "He who has a *why* to live for, can bear with almost any *how*." (*Man's Search For Meaning,* N.Y.: Washington Square Press, 1963, p. 121). During his conversations with the three friends, Job contended that if he knew the *why* of his calamities, he could endure them. After his encounter with God in the whirlwind, Job still does not know *why,* but he can live with it. The reason: he knows the *Who*. He who knows the *Who* can bear with any *how,* even though he knows not the *why.* Trust in the *Who* brings security even to those without answers. It is one thing to hear of God by the hearing of the ear; it is another to see him with the eyes of faith. Only then can we *know*.

5. Knowing—A Phenomenon of Both Brains

Such *knowing* depends on the involvement of both of our brains, the left brain with its focus on reason and the right brain with its focus on intuition. When pummeled by God's hard-hitting questions, Job's left brain was beaten into submission. He obviously had no answers. After God continued to question, Job's right brain became involved. Behind the rational and persistent questioning, Job perceived—or intuited—a caring questioner. Then Job's submission in the first part of the theophany became his affirmation of faith in the second. After the first part, God was all transcendent might; after the second, God was also imminent and caring. The God of power and might is also the God of love, and our inner door of consciousness, our right brain, needs to know this.

In his *Answer to Job* (Hull, N.Y.: Pastoral Psychology Book Club, 1955), psychoanalyst Carl Jung says that Job had the best of the argument. He received no reason from God for his sufferings that would justify them. His left brain—reason—was left unsatisfied. On the basis of left-brain logic, Job won the contest. God knows this, says Jung, even though Job is reconciled with his pain. In fact, with tongue in cheek, Jung says that God feels badly—even guilty—about this "victory." So God has the need to enter the human scene of suffering—to become incarnate in human flesh. In Christ, God endures this suffering to the same excruciating level, and in the cry of dereliction from the cross, he asks the Jobian question, why? Why, God? "My God, my God, why hast thou forsaken me?" (Mk. 15:34).

God's empathy is an empathy of *identification*. God knows Job's agony because in Jesus the Christ, God has been there. God's answer to Job is in the incarnation, when God became Job, and in so doing, God became the mediator for whom Job longed. While God did not let Job die of his sufferings, even though he longed for death, Jesus died from his. And then God raised him from the dead. In *this* victory, God led Jesus beyond "songs in the night" to the dawn of a new day. This then is the ultimate answer to Job, and to every one of us who suffers.

6. A Retroactive Evaluation

How, in retrospect, can we evaluate the spiritual counseling of the three friends of Job? Despite all of their emotional reaction to Job, in which they went from the defensive to the offensive, they did not drop the subject. They got the despondent Job so involved in his combat with them that in the end he was more angry than depressed. They only gave up when Job systematically and totally rejected their premise and approach.

Elihu was the transitional person who took Job off the defensive, identified with him, and allowed his suffering to be free of judgment. He shared a vision of redemption for Job which could give him hope, but he himself could not bring that redemption about. Elihu prepared the way for Job to receive the One who could bring it about. He prepared the way for Job to see God.

In St. Paul's metaphor for ministry, the three friends, despite how poorly they went about it, were sowers and waterers. This was as far as they could go. Elihu, also a sower and waterer, sensed his limits more than the three friends, and after he finished what he could do, he asked Job to join him in awaiting the One who could "give the growth" (1 Cor. 3:6–7).

In a broad sense these counselors also were mediators—as we who counsel are mediators—who bring the troubled to the One mediator for whom they, like Job, long—the man Christ Jesus, through whom we see God (John 14:8–10; 1 Tim. 2:5).

EPILOGUE

The epilogue, chapter 42:7–17, returns to the prose style of the prologue. As in the prologue Job's possessions are taken from him, so in the epilogue they are restored. In fact, he received "twice as much as he had before . . . fourteen thousand sheep, six thousand camels, a thousand yoke of oxen, and a thousand she-asses" (42:10, 12). He also had only seven new sons and three new daughters, presumably by the wife mentioned in the prologue.

In addition, "Then came to him all his brothers and sisters and all who had known him before, ate bread with him in his house, and they showed him sympathy and comforted him for all the evil that the Lord had brought upon him; and each of them gave him a piece of money and a ring of gold" (42:11). These were the people who found him repulsive while he was still in his agony and turned away from him (12:4; 16:20; 19:17). Job's graciousness is shown in his receiving them and welcoming them back. Job himself got to see the longevity he had anticipated prior to his calamities fulfilled (29:18). "And after this Job lived a hundred and forty years, and saw his sons, and his sons' sons, four generations. And Job died, an old man, and full of days" (42:16–17).

1. A Completing of the Story

Does the epilogue pose a problem? After Job's experience of *knowing*, in which he found his songs in the midst of the night, the restoration of his material, physical, and familial blessings seems anticlimatic. Does it seem that someone who had not appreciated the fulfillment in Job's songs in the night thought the book needed a happy ending? Perhaps—if one sees in the epilogue only the blessings restored, and not that

116

Job is now a different person. Even in this restoration, the meaning of his possessions is different than before. He has learned to be content with God's favor, even without them. Actually, the epilogue completes the drama of the prologue; the purpose for Job's sufferings had been accomplished. The restoration of Job's losses is the coherent consequence of the drama's completion. In a sense, this restoration of losses is symbolic of the restoration of Job himself—with spiritual blessings that he had not known before (42:5).

2. Symbol of the Resurrection

Like the "songs in the night," the restoration of blessings can also be looked upon as a symbol of the resurrection. Job had his songs in the night; now he has his songs in the day. As his spirit was resurrected from his sense of alienation from God in his songs in the night, his seeing God included seeing the eternal dimensions of life in the here and now. His songs in the day, then, symbolized the eschatological fulfillment of this seeing—where there shall be no more pain or crying (Rev. 21:4). Since Job on more than one occasion raised not only the question but also the hope and the vision of life that transcends physical death, the symbolic purpose of these songs in the night and in the day fits into the restoration of the epilogue.

3. Changes in Job's Relationships with Others

In the epilogue, the changes in Job go beyond those in his spirit, described in his second response to God in the theophany, to those of his actions in regard to his fellow human beings. Changes in our system with God lead to changes in our system with ourself and to our systems with others. In addition to welcoming back his brothers, sisters and friends, his relationship with the three friends also needed mending. While they may have had it with Job, God had it with them. In order to bring about their reconciliation, they are directed by God to make the traditional sacrifice of rams and bulls, and then Job would pray for their forgiveness. But the emphasis in their reconciliation is on Job's prayer of intercession. In response to Job's prayer, God promises to "accept his prayer not to deal with you (the friends) according to your folly" (42:8). The three friends did as they were told, and God accepted Job's prayer.

In the prologue, Job's sons and daughters are not named, but in the epilogue the *daughters* alone are named. This is highly unusual for the patriarchal era. But what is more unusual is that Job gave them inheritance among their brothers. For Job, their being women did not make them less important to his posterity than their brothers. In Old Testament times, daughters were usually allowed inheritance only when there were no sons.

4. Significant Omissions

There is no mention of Elihu in the epilogue. However, the purpose of the epilogue is unfinished business. The three friends are mentioned because of the need for their reconciliation and forgiveness. There is no such need for Elihu. His relationship with Job simply faded out as his words prepared the way for Job's encounter with God.

Nor is there any mention in the epilogue of the *why* of Job's sufferings. The drama of the prologue between God and Satan is not mentioned. Consequently, Job never received his *why,* even in the restoration of his blessings. It had become irrelevant.